Hypertrophic Cardiomyopathy

Hypertrophic Cardiomyopathy
A Practical Guide to Diagnosis and Management

Edited By
Srilakshmi M. Adhyapak
V. Rao Parachuri

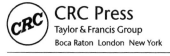

CRC Press
Taylor & Francis Group
Boca Raton London New York

CRC Press is an imprint of the
Taylor & Francis Group, an **informa** business

First edition published 2021
by CRC Press
6000 Broken Sound Parkway NW, Suite 300, Boca Raton, FL 33487-2742

and by CRC Press
2 Park Square, Milton Park, Abingdon, Oxon, OX14 4RN

© 2021 Taylor & Francis Group, LLC

CRC Press is an imprint of Taylor & Francis Group, LLC

Library of Congress Cataloging-in-Publication Data

A catalog record has been requested for this book

ISBN: 978-0-367-56804-7 (hbk)
ISBN: 978-0-429-33034-6 (ebk)

Typeset in Minion
by SPi Global, India

Visit the Supplementary Material: www.routledge.com/9780367352813

DEDICATION

This book is dedicated to all the scientists, researchers, students, anatomists, physiologists, cardiologists, and cardiac surgeons who have spent their lives seeking to understand the various presentations of hypertrophic cardiomyopathy, which encompasses a whole clinical syndrome in itself. The book is also dedicated to those who have spent their lives seeking to evolve innovations that tackle and reverse the relentless downhill course of this condition.

CONTENTS

FOREWORD

The description and recognition of hypertrophic cardiomyopathy (HCM) has undergone considerable evolution over the past six decades, when there has been an increase in awareness, including diagnostic acumen, requiring the development of dedicated multidisciplinary HCM centers. The developments in diagnostic tools have shed light on the change in epidemiology of HCM. It is now known to include patients from a wide variety of races, cultures, ethnicities, and both sexes – equally.

The occurrence of HCM can be attributed to spontaneous (*de novo*) mutations among 11 genes encoding thick and thin filament proteins of the cardiac sarcomere (most commonly the beta-myosin heavy chain) and the myosin-binding protein C. Estimates of the prevalence of HCM have been reported disproportionately, the prevalence being higher in developed countries with advanced medical systems. An occurrence as high as 1:500 has been reported in the general population based on clinical expression of the disease's phenotype, which is left ventricular hypertrophy, evidenced by imaging. A more recent higher estimate of 1:200 took into account a broader clinical profile based on familial transmission and contemporary imaging, as well as the high frequency of pathogenic sarcomere gene mutations which are known to occur in the affected population. The prevalence is not clearly known in developing countries where there are significant numbers of patients who go unrecognized. Due to sudden cardiac death being a manifestation of disease, many patients go undetected. This further emphasizes the need for early detection and treatment of this condition, predicating the need for multi-disciplinary teams and centers in these countries.

Surgical myectomy is currently advocated for obstructive HCM in patients with disabling heart failure (symptoms classified as New York Heart Association [NYHA] class III/IV), which has to be refractory to anti-heart failure medications, per the American Heart Association/American College of Cardiology/European Society of Cardiology expert consensus guidelines.

This requirement of symptoms refractory to maximally tolerated medications as a prerequisite for surgery was largely influenced by the prohibitive mortality rates of myectomy of 8% nearly three decades ago. Of late, there are several surgeons and cardiologists who feel a compelling need to revise this treatment strategy to include patients who are less symptomatic (in NYHA class II) but with symptoms significantly impacting their quality of life. The thought of calling for revision of the present guidelines has resulted from observational studies demonstrating a substantial reduction in operative mortality for HCM, including the apical and mid-ventricular obstructive type, from 8% to 0.4% (a nearly 95% magnitude decrease).

Myectomy has been shown to reverse heart failure symptoms. It has also been shown to decrease the incidence of sudden death and obviate the need for intracardiac defibrillator (ICD) implantations in a few anecdotal reports. Nearly 90% of patients have shown improvement in heart failure symptoms following myectomy, with 70% having no residual symptoms when resuming normal activity (NYHA class I).

The problems facing HCM surgery, as observed by Dr Joseph Dearani, is that patients worldwide with hypertrophic obstructive cardiomyopathy do not receive optimal treatment. Patients are either kept on medical therapy (despite symptoms), referred for a less effective intervention (alcohol septal ablation), or undergo suboptimal and unnecessarily dangerous (as great as 6% mortality!) septal myectomies by surgeons who are not experienced in this field. One of the problems is the misconception that septal myectomy is a very simple procedure.

Surgeons do need to learn a few careful steps regarding the surgical procedure, as well as to know the precise anatomic indications that must often be tailored to the individual, and to assess whether the patient will indeed benefit from a myectomy operation.

Lack of this knowledge leads to a vicious cycle with patients receiving suboptimal surgery, negative clinical results, fewer referrals by cardiologists to surgery, thereby reducing surgical experience further, with deterioration of outcomes – thus perpetuating the cycle.

The only way to break this vicious cycle is to create a worldwide network of mentors who will define the appropriate centers where there is a solid team composed of hypertrophic obstructive cardiomyopathy cardiologists and interested cardiac surgeons, to help train and evolve a center of excellence.

I am personally indebted to my colleague surgeon Dr P. V. Rao for creating a "center for hypertrophic cardiomyopathy" at NH health city in Bangalore by performing nearly 300 septal myectomies for obstruction at all levels. Many young surgeons trained at this center are performing septal myectomies across the country with excellent results. The management of HCM requires a team approach, especially the support of imaging for optimal myectomy. I acknowledge the contributions of Dr Vimal Raj and Dr Satish Govind in this context.

I would like to congratulate Dr Srilakshmi for the excellent work done in compiling this book with contributions from some of the pioneers in this field.

Dr Devi Shetty MS, FRCS (England)
Chairman, Narayana Health
Bangalore

PREFACE

The goal of this book is to provide cardiac surgeons and cardiologists with a comprehensive perspective of the clinicopathological entity of hypertrophic cardiomyopathy (HCM). This, in its early stages, is amenable to medical therapy, but when its symptoms become refractory to medical therapy, surgical myectomy becomes the cornerstone of treatment.

The objective of this book therefore is to discuss the various aspects of this unique disease with special emphasis on the surgical techniques for an optimal myectomy which should result in near physiological hemodynamics being evident over the long term. Due to the steep learning curve that exists for this procedure, our aim was to discuss the unique features of this disease and to attempt a surgical guide for optimal myectomy. The treatment has been aptly described as "the knife which heals," referring to the American College of Cardiology/American Heart Association (ACC/AHA) recommendations of myectomy as being the gold standard for treatment of HCM.

Surgical techniques are an evolution refined by masters in the field; and in the case of myectomy it was begun by William Cleland.

In 1958 Cleland first performed a myectomy for HCM with a left ventricular outflow obstruction. Andrew Morrow, James Kirklin, and Wilfred Gordon Bigelow subsequently contributed extensively to the evolution of this procedure. Recently, several modifications and refinements have been devised for the different phenotypes of this entity. Dr Hartzel Schaff and others at the Mayo Clinic have contributed extensively toward myectomy for the various HCM phenotypes. Dr Parachuri, who has co authored Chapter 6, was a cardiac surgical trainee at Harefield hospital, London during the late eighties and had the opportunity to witness Prof Sir Magdi Yacoub perform myectomy in his own masterly way. This was the beginning of Parachuri's interest in surgery for HCM, culminating in the present book. The surgical steps of myectomy have been explained lucidly in a video linked to Chapter 6 (https://www.routledge.com/9780367352813).

This book highlights the need for a team approach to the management of this disease, one which involves cardiologists, cardiac surgeons, radiologists, geneticists, and counselors.

Srilakshmi M. Adhyapak
Bangalore, India
V. Rao Parachuri
Bangalore, India

ACKNOWLEDGMENTS

We wish to express our thanks to all the authors of the various chapters. We also wish to express our thanks to all the authors and publishers who permitted us to quote their publications, figures, and data in this book. We wish to specially thank Dr Devi Prasad Shetty at Narayana Hrudayalaya Institute of Medical Sciences, Bangalore, for his constant encouragement. Finally, we wish to thank the editorial and production staff at Taylor & Francis for their professional help and cooperation in producing this book.

EDITORS

Dr V. Rao Parachuri FRCS (CTh) started his medical career at Madras Medical College. He later trained at Hammersmith and Harefield Hospitals, UK and worked as a fellow at St. Vincent Hospital, Worcester, Massachusetts, USA. His field of interest is in the surgical management of heart failure with special interest in myectomy for hypertrophic cardiomyopathy. He has performed over 300 surgical myectomy procedures. His other interests include mitral and aortic valve repairs, surgical ventricular restoration, and surgical pulmonary vein isolation for atrial fibrillation. He has performed nearly 500 surgical ventricular restoration operations and over 25,000 coronary artery bypass grafts (CABGs) and valve repairs. He is Senior Consultant Cardiac Surgeon at Narayana Hrudayalaya Institute of Medical Sciences, Bangalore, India. He has nearly 50 publications to his credit and has co-authored a book on surgical ventricular restoration.

Dr Srilakshmi M. Adhyapak DNB trained in interventional cardiology at Narayana Hrudayalaya Institute of Medical Sciences, Bangalore, India. Her interests are in heart failure and various interventions directed at halting its progress. She is presently Associate Professor of Cardiology at St. John's Medical College Hospital, Bangalore, India. She has nearly 50 publications to her credit and two books.

CONTRIBUTORS

Dr Hashim Ahamed DM
Department of Cardiology
Amritha Institute of Medical Sciences
Kochi, India

Dr Gulhane Avanti MD
Department of Cardiovascular Imaging
University of Pennsylvania
Philadelphia, Pennsylvania, USA

Dr Vinay Badhwar MD
Department of Cardiovascular and Thoracic
    Surgery
West Virginia University
Morgantown, West Virginia, USA

Dr Sreekar Balasundaram DNB
Department of Cardiothoracic Surgery
St. John's Medical College Hospital
Bangalore, India

Dr Milind Y. Desai MD
Department of Cardiology
Cleveland Clinic
Cleveland, Ohio, USA

Dr Satish C. Govind MD
Department of Echocardiography
Narayana Hrudayalaya
Bangalore, India

Dr Heather K. Hayanga
Division of Cardiovascular and Thoracic
    Anesthesiology
West Virginia University
Morgantown, West Virginia, USA

Dr Jeremiah W. Hayanga
Department of Cardiovascular and
    Thoracic Surgery
West Virginia University
Morgantown, West Virginia, USA

Dr Kevin Hodges
Department of Cardiothoracic Surgery
Cleveland Medical Center
Cleveland, Ohio, USA

Dr Ameya Kaskar
Department of Cardiac Surgery
Narayana Hrudayalaya Institute of
    Medical Sciences
Bangalore, India

Joseph McGuire
West Virginia University School of
    Medicine
Morgantown, West Virginia, USA

Dr Prahlad G. Menon PhD
Department of Biomedical Engineering
University of Pittsburgh

and

Department of Mathematics &
    Data Analytics
Carlow University
Pittsburgh, Pennsylvania, USA

Dr Nicholas Smedira
Department of Cardiothoracic Surgery
Cleveland Medical Center
Cleveland, Ohio, USA

Dr Paul Sorajja MD
Department of Cardiology
Minneapolis Heart Institute
Rochester, Minnesota, USA

Dr Charlotte Spear MD
Department of Cardiovascular and Thoracic
    Surgery
West Virginia University
Morgantown, West Virginia, USA

Dr Anene C. Ukaigwe
Center for Valve and Structural Heart
    Disease
Minneapolis Heart Institute Foundation
Minneapolis Heart Institute at Abbott
    Northwestern Hospital
Minneapolis, Minnesota, USA

Dr Raj Vimal MD
Department of Radiology
Narayana Hrudayalaya
Bangalore, India

Dr Tom Kai Ming Wang
Section of Cardiovascular Imaging
Heart and Vascular Institute
Cleveland Clinic
Cleveland, Ohio, USA

Dr Lawrence M. Wei MD
Department of Cardiovascular and Thoracic
    Surgery
West Virginia University
Morgantown, West Virginia, USA

Dr Per Wierup MD
Department of Cardiac Surgery
Cleveland Clinic
Cleveland, Ohio, USA

Dr Lakhani Zeeshan MD
Department of Radiology
NH Health City
Bangalore, India

Chapter 1

HYPERTROPHIC CARDIOMYOPATHY
An Overview

Srilakshmi M. Adhyapak

CONTENTS

INTRODUCTION

PREVALENCE

The prevalence of hypertrophic cardiomyopathy (HCM) has been reported as 1:500, with greater prevalence noted recently [1]. The earliest reports of it were largely limited to developed countries of North America and Western Europe in Caucasians, but shortly thereafter there were reports of it from Japan, which helped the compilation of a substantial literature on it in Asians [2]. With enhanced awareness and diagnostic acumen, and the development of dedicated multidisciplinary centers [1], the epidemiology of HCM has evolved to include patients from a wide variety of races, cultures, ethnicities, and both sexes – equally (see Figure 1.1). The occurrence of HCM can be attributed to spontaneous (*de novo*) mutations among 11 genes

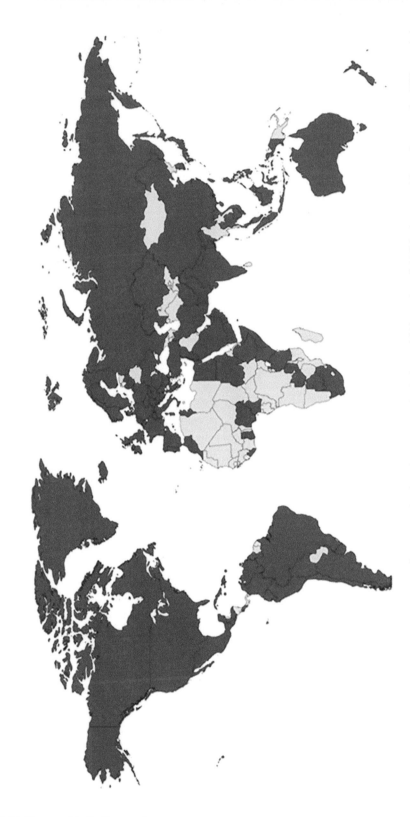

Figure 1.1 World map showing global distribution of HCM, which is found in 122 countries in the world (shown in red). HCM = hypertrophic cardiomyopathy. With permission of B.J. Maron et al., "Global Burden of Hypertrophic Cardiomyopathy." *JACC: Heart Failure* (2018) 6: 376–378.

encoding thick and thin filament proteins of the cardiac sarcomere (most commonly the beta-myosin heavy chain and myosin-binding protein C). Estimates of the prevalence of HCM have been reported disproportionately from developed countries with advanced medical systems. An occurrence of 1:500 in the general population has been reported based on clinical expression of the disease's phenotype, which is left ventricular hypertrophy, evidenced by imaging. A more recent higher estimate of 1:200 takes into account a broader clinical profile based on familial transmission and contemporary imaging, as well as the high frequency of pathogenic sarcomere gene mutations which are known to occur in the affected population [3].

CLINICAL FEATURES AND PRESENTATION
Diagnosis of HCM is often challenging due to its phenotypic heterogeneity. In a majority of diagnosed patients, prognosis is generally favorable, with sudden cardiac death (SCD) and severe congestive heart failure occurring only in a subset of patients. Treatment is multifaceted, requiring individualized care. The clinical presentation has morphed from SCD to heart failure with the advent of implantable cardioverter defibrillators (ICD), which have substantially decreased the incidence of SCD, making heart failure increasingly prevalent [2].

Hypertrophic cardiomyopathy-related heart failure differs from heart failure by other causes. Heart failure as manifested by exertional dyspnea ranges in severity from mild to severe (New York Heart Association [NYHA] functional classes II to IV), the progression of which becomes refractory to medical management, leading to progressive disability, though occurring largely in the absence of pulmonary congestion and volume overload. HCM-related heart failure is most commonly due to dynamic mechanical impedance to left ventricular outflow produced by mitral valve systolic anterior motion, leading to high intracavity pressures. Traditionally recognized as heart failure, exertional dyspnea is the most prominent cause of functional disability in HCM.

HYPERTROPHIC CARDIOMYOPATHY PHENOTYPES AND THEIR CLINICAL PRESENTATION
A wall thickness of $\geq$ 15 mm by echocardiography, computed tomography, or cardiac magnetic resonance (CMR) in the absence of a secondary cause for hypertrophy is consistent with HCM [2]. Left ventricular hypertrophy (LVH) typically manifests as asymmetric septal hypertrophy, reminiscent of its early description by Braunwald et al. as idiopathic hypertrophy of the interventricular septum. Advanced imaging techniques have increased awareness of other patterns of hypertrophy, namely, apical, concentric, lateral wall, and right ventricular. In first-degree family members of patients with unequivocal disease, an unexplained wall thickness of $\geq$ 13 mm is sufficient for diagnosis [3]. Electron microscopy and CMR imaging have identified myofibrillar disarray and extensive late gadolinium enhancement on CMR, defining fibrosis as accompanying findings. Diastolic dysfunction in HCM is ubiquitous and secondary to hemodynamic derangements, including prolonged and non-uniform ventricular relaxation, loss of ventricular suction, decreased chamber compliance, and abnormal intracellular calcium uptake [4].

HYPERTROPHIC OBSTRUCTIVE CARDIOMYOPATHY
Dynamic left ventricular outflow tract (LVOT) obstruction, defined as LVOT gradient $\geq$ 30 mm Hg [5], is a determinant of a therapeutic approach to HCM. Approximately 70% of HCM patients have LVOT obstruction at rest or with provocation.

Subaortic obstruction or LVOT obstruction is usually due to mitral valve systolic anterior motion with septal contact, facilitated by the hydrodynamic force of flow drag (Figure 1.2). Additional morphologic abnormalities, including elongated mitral valve leaflets, abnormally positioned and hypertrophied papillary muscles, and accessory LV muscle bundles, may also contribute to the mechanism of outflow obstruction. Mechanical impedance due to subaortic obstruction results in LV systolic pressure overload associated with secondary mild-to-moderate mitral regurgitation and preserved or increased (hyperdynamic) LV function [6]. In about 5% of HCM cases, obstruction occurs in the mid-ventricle by muscular apposition of the septum and anomalous anterolateral papillary muscle inserting directly

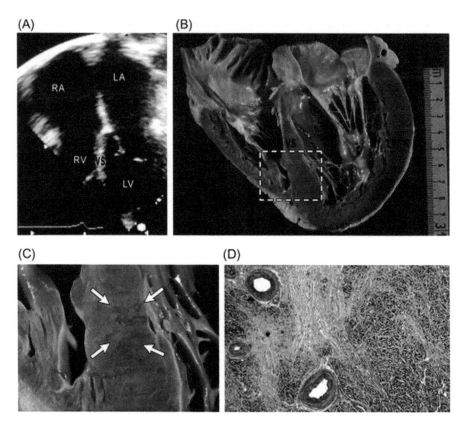

Figure 1.2 End-stage systolic dysfunction. A 59-year-old transplanted male patient with a tro-ponin T mutation. (*A*) Four-chamber view at end-diastole showing dilatation of both atria (trans-verse left atrial [LV] dimension = 70 mm), left ventricular (LV) enlargement (i.e., 62 mm), and mild hypertrophy (septal ventricular septum [VS] thickness; 13 mm); ejection fraction (EF) was 30%. (*B*) Heart removed at transplantation. Note thinning of the basal and mid-ventricular septum (12 mm) compared with distal LV. (*C*) High power of boxed area shown in (*B*). Grayish areas (arrows) are indicative of septal scarring. (*D*) Area of the septum shown in (*C*). Extensive replacement fibrosis is associated with abnormal intramural arterioles. Trichrome stain ×60. RA, right atrium; RV, right ventricle. With permission of Paola Melacini et al., "Clinicopathological Profiles of Progressive Heart Failure in Hypertrophic Cardiomyopathy." *European Heart Journal* (2010) 31, 2111–2123.

into the anterior leaflet, or septal, and LV free wall contact in patients with LV apical aneu-rysms [7]. Outflow obstruction in HCM is notable for spontaneous variability, often day to day or even hourly, explaining why mild rest gradients (30 to 49 mm Hg) are associated with the same risk of development of heart failure symptoms as are higher rest gradients (≥ 70 mm Hg) [8]. Obstruction can also be triggered by physiological loading changes, such as standing, hydration, meals, or alcohol consumption, or any variable that enhances LV contractility and cardiac output, such as tachycardia or reduced ventricular volume [6]. Some symptoms are less explainable in HCM, especially the variability of presentation. Some patients tolerate outflow obstruction with stability over long periods of time, extend-ing into advanced ages without symptoms, while others require intervention in childhood or as young adults [9]. Although elevated LV systolic pressures (and mitral regurgitation) rep-resent the primary triggers for exertional dyspnea, its pathophysiology is likely to be multi-factorial with contributing and interrelated mechanisms: impaired LV filling (evident by elevated end-diastolic pressure), impaired stroke volume/cardiac output with exercise [10], left atrial and pulmonary hypertension, and microvascular ischemia [11–14]. The precise contribution of these variables to symptoms remains unresolved due to limited invasive hemodynamic and metabolic studies focused on the mechanism and the lack of suitable HCM animal models. The mechanism by which pulmonary hypertension occurs in HCM is incompletely resolved, although increased LV systolic and end-diastolic cavity pressures due to obstruction (and mitral regurgitation) can secondarily increase the left atrial and pulmonary artery pressure [15]. Pulmonary hypertension in HCM is not a contra-indication for myectomy and does not increase risk during septal myectomy. In many patients, following myectomy, pulmonary pressures tend to decrease (or normalize) [15].

NON-OBSTRUCTIVE HCM

Patients who do not generate outflow gradients at rest or with physiological (exercise) provocation comprise about one-third of patients with HCM [16]. Most non-obstructive patients commonly have a relatively benign or stable clinical course with mild heart failure (HF) symptoms, but uncommonly (about 10%) progress to severe limitation and disability refractory to maximal medical management [10, 17, 18]. Such end-stage patients in NYHA functional class III/IV comprise 2% to 3% [18] and demonstrate a unique phenotypic transformation from diastolic dysfunction to LV systolic pump failure with systolic dysfunction (Figure 1.2). There occurs LV remodeling comprising wall thinning and/or ventricular chamber enlargement due to diffuse myocardial scarring [4, 19, 20].

APICAL HCM

This abnormal phenotype was initially described in Japan by Sakamoto et al. and later by Yamaguchi et al. These patients present with predominant hypertrophy of the apex, leading to a diminished ventricular cavity size. This was initially discovered when the resting electrocardiogram (ECG) demonstrated deep T wave inversions in the precordial leads, and the left ventricular cine-angiography demonstrated apical obliteration with spade-like configuration of the apex. Outside Asia, the prevalence is < 1%. These patients have a relatively benign course while some present early due to LV diastolic dysfunction. They become refractory to medical therapy earlier than the obstructive and non-obstructive phenotypes. Due to the abnormal LV cavity shape and size, other options for refractory heart failure such as left ventricular assist device implantation are not feasible [7]. Myectomy in these patients has shown good results.

HYPERTROPHIC CARDIOMYOPATHY WITH PRESERVED LEFT VENTRICLE FUNCTION AND ADVANCED HEART FAILURE

Extensive heterogeneity exists within a relatively small end-stage subset, as paradoxically 50% of patients with refractory symptoms demonstrate preserved systolic function (EF ≥ 50%) [19]. This under-recognized HCM phenotype is characterized by modest LV remodeling with normal (or small) cavity size, no or minimal myocardial fibrosis, but impaired cardiac output and LV filling [19] (Figures 1.3–1.5). Notably, the profile of this subgroup with HCM and preserved EF resembles patients with conventional cardiac failure and preserved EF.

ROLE OF IMAGING IN HCM

Trans-thoracic echocardiography remains the mainstay of cardiac imaging in HCM, requiring an organized and detailed assessment.

Demonstration of the severity and distribution of LVH is vital to diagnosis and management of HCM. The severity of LVH is important in prognostication and SCD risk assessment. A stepwise increase in SCD risk is associated with increasing wall thickness, with a cutoff of ≥ 30 mm considered as "massive" hypertrophy.

Abnormalities of the mitral valve and mitral apparatus are common in HCM, with leaflets longer than those in control patients, independent of wall thickness or mass index [7]. Numerous papillary muscle abnormalities have been described, chief of them being a direct insertion of the valve leaflet into the papillary muscle [21].

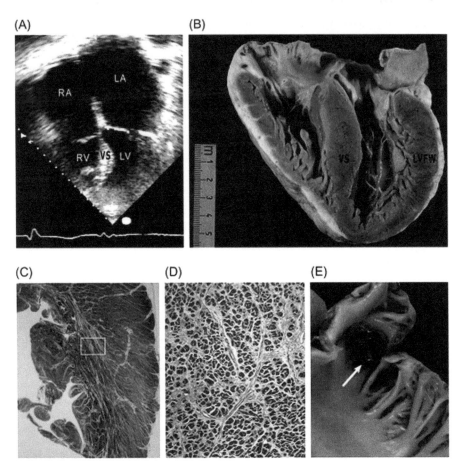

Figure 1.3 Non-obstructive hypertrophic cardiomyopathy with preserved systolic function (and atrial fibrillation). A 60-year-old male patient with a β-myosin heavy chain mutation. (*A*) Four-chamber view at end-diastole showing severe dilatation of both atria (transverse dimension of left atrium [LA], 90 mm), normal-sized left ventricle (LV) and right ventricle (RV), and mild LV hypertrophy (ventricular septum, VS; 18 mm) as well as preserved systolic function. (*B*) Heart removed at transplantation. (*C*) Histological section of left ventricular free wall (LVFW) showing the absence of replacement fibrosis. Trichrome stain ×3. (*D*) High-power view of the area in box in (*C*) showing increased interstitial fibrosis. Trichrome stain ×40. (*E*) Thrombus within LA appendage (arrow). RA, right atrium. With permission of Paola Melacini et al., "Clinicopathological Profiles of Progressive Heart Failure in Hypertrophic Cardiomyopathy." *European Heart Journal* (2010) 31, 2111–2123.

In LVOT obstruction, mitral valve systolic anterior motion (SAM) produces a dynamic, eccentric, posteriorly directed jet of regurgitation. Other mechanisms of regurgitation must be considered when the jet is not posteriorly directed.

A systematic approach to provocation of LVOT obstruction should be used. Obstruction can occur at the mid-ventricular level or can be at multiple levels (both at LVOT and mid-ventricular levels) [10].

Myocardial strain imaging adds to the characterization of HCM. Characterization of diastolic strain, including quantization of untwist, may provide further insight into abnormalities of diastolic filling in HCM [13]. The quantization of untwist at the apex is particularly affected in HCM, unlike in LVH, due to other causes.

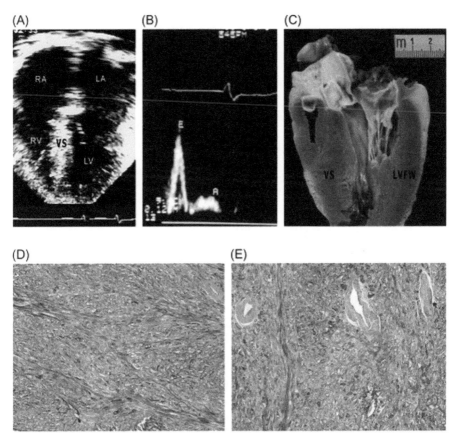

Figure 1.4 Non-obstructive hypertrophic cardiomyopathy with preserved systolic function. Restrictive form of heart failure due to diastolic dysfunction in sinus rhythm. A 28-year-old woman with troponin I mutation. (A) Four-chamber view in end-diastole showing dilatation of both atria (left atrium, LA = 53 mm), normal-sized ventricles, and mild ventricular septal (VS) thickening (17 mm). (B) Pulsed Doppler waveform with evidence of restrictive filling: E/A > 2; deceleration time < 150 ms. (C) Long-axis left ventricular (LV) plane with mild VS hypertrophy (17 mm); atria missing due to transplantation. (D and E) LV free wall (D) and septum (E) showing diffuse myocardial disarray, mild interstitial fibrosis, and intramural small vessel disease. Trichrome stain ×40. LVFW, left ventricular free wall; RA, right atrium; RV, right ventricle. With permission of Paola Melacini et al., "Clinicopathological Profiles of Progressive Heart Failure in Hypertrophic Cardiomyopathy." *European Heart Journal* (2010) 31, 2111–2123.

CARDIAC MAGNETIC RESONANCE IMAGING

Cardiac magnetic resonance (CMR) has definite advantages over echocardiography, with superior spatial resolution and accurate volumetric assessment of all cardiac chambers. The images are independent of the body habitus, chest wall geometry, and pulmonary parenchymal disease, which limit echocardiographic acoustic windows. However, the image quality in CMR is dependent upon cardiac and respiratory gating, with a need for prolonged breath hold for some image sequences.

The greatest additive value of CMR for HCM is tissue characterization. Sequences such as myocardial nulling and T2 assessment help exclude similar phenotype cardiac conditions like cardiac amyloidosis and hemochromatosis. Late gadolinium enhancement (LGE) sequences provide *in vivo* definition of myocardial fibrosis. Extensive LGE predicts an

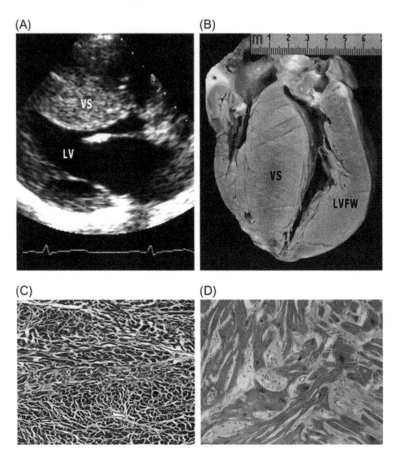

Figure 1.5 Non-obstructive hypertrophic cardiomyopathy with preserved systolic function. A 12-year-old girl with massive septal hypertrophy in sinus rhythm with a myosin-binding protein-C mutation. (A) Parasternal long-axis view at end-diastole, showing marked septal hypertrophy (30 mm) and normal-sized left ventricular (LV) cavity. (B) Explanted heart, showing massive asymmetric hypertrophy of ventricular septum (VS), and absence of grossly visible scars. (C and D) Sections of left ventricular free wall (LVFW) (C) and VS (D) showing myocyte hypertrophy and disarray, and increased interstitial fibrosis. Trichrome stain, ×20 and ×40. With permission of Paola Melacini et al., "Clinicopathological Profiles of Progressive Heart Failure in Hypertrophic Cardiomyopathy." *European Heart Journal* (2010) 31, 2111–2123.

adverse prognosis in HCM, with multiple studies demonstrating correlations with increased wall thickness, exercise test evidence of ischemia, reduction in ejection fraction, nonsustained ventricular tachycardia (VT), and mortality. The presence of > 15% LGE is a predictor of SCD in HCM.

RISK OF SUDDEN CARDIAC DEATH (SCD)

Patients with HCM and prior cardiac arrest should undergo ICD insertion. For primary prevention, one accessible approach to risk stratification is the HCM Risk-SCD calculator that incorporates age, extent of LVH, left atrium size, LVOT gradient, family history of SCD, nonsustained VT, and unexplained syncope to predict five-year SCD risk [9].

American Heart Association/American College of Cardiology (ACCF/AHA) guidelines heavily emphasize that the risk of SCD is associated with massive hypertrophy, unexplained syncope, and family history of SCD, stating a class IIa recommendation for ICD insertion in these patients [2]. Even though these extensive guidelines are available to guide therapy, clinical judgment remains paramount.

PREDICTORS OF HEART FAILURE

Hypertrophic cardiomyopathy, when symptomatic, carries a grave prognosis. With the known peculiarities in heart failure in HCM patients, it is worthwhile screening such patients for impending heart failure.

EXERCISE (STRESS) ECHOCARDIOGRAPHY

Combining echocardiography with exercise testing is the most reliable method for provoking dynamic physiological LV outflow gradients in patients without obstruction at rest, and has attained an important role in surveillance of patients with HCM [16]. This test non-invasively identifies the subgroup of HCM patients with capacity to generate significant impedance to LV outflow solely with exercise provocation and, in the process, resolves the differential diagnosis of obstructive versus non-obstructive HCM [16, 18]. This is of particular clinical relevance in severely limited patients (NYHA functional class III/IV) with exercise-provoked outflow gradients who can be candidates for septal reduction intervention, whereas an inability to generate obstruction with exercise (or at rest) confines management options to heart transplantation after these patients have become refractory to medical therapy [18].

Stress echocardiography predicts the future risk for developing advanced symptoms in asymptomatic (or mildly symptomatic) patients. Patients with physiologically provoked obstruction are at risk of developing advanced HF symptoms at 3.2% per year, compared with only 1.6% per year for non-obstructive patients [18].

METABOLIC (CARDIOPULMONARY) TESTING

Peak myocardial oxygen consumption (VO_2), assessed by cardiopulmonary exercise testing (CPET), is a reproducible measure of functional capacity. In HCM, peak VO_2 is reduced in most symptomatic patients, correlating with NYHA functional class [12, 13, 21]. Assessment of disabling symptoms and related management decisions in HCM are made predominantly with traditional history taking, in accordance with the expert consensus guidelines [2, 3]. For most patients with obstructive HCM, CPET does not significantly impact management decisions unless the level of disability is ambiguous on history taking and cannot be assessed reliably.

Cardiopulmonary exercise testing is a conventional component of the targeted heart transplant evaluation in non-obstructive HCM, with peak $VO_2 \leq 14$ ml/kg/min (or $\leq 50\%$ predicted for age) being an important metric in determining candidacy [22]. However, patients who fail to achieve this traditional cutoff should not be excluded from transplant consideration solely on this basis because some patients with HCM demonstrate a mismatch between peak VO_2 and severe exercise limitation [19].

BIOMARKERS

Brain natriuretic peptide (or N-terminal pro-brain natriuretic peptide), although useful in non-HCM patient populations, is not a reliable predictor of outcome for individual patients with HCM [23]. The severity of heart failure in HCM is familial. End-stage HF can cluster in some families so that its occurrence in one family member increases the risk for others [19, 20].

LIFESTYLE MEASURES

Participation in competitive sports is discouraged by the guidelines [2]. Avoidance of excess alcohol or stimulant consumption, dehydration, and temperature extremes (e.g., saunas and hot tubs) are recommended. Use of phosphodiesterase inhibitors for erectile dysfunction may result in hemodynamic instability in the setting of LVOT obstruction, and therefore caution is advised.

DRUGS

Traditional pharmacological strategies to control or reduce exertional symptoms in HCM have been largely empiric, based on retrospective observational studies [1–3, 24, 25]. Drug treatment has consisted primarily of beta blockers and calcium antagonists (predominantly verapamil) [25], which improve LV filling but do not significantly reduce outflow gradients at rest. There is no evidence that aldosterone antagonist drugs (e.g., spironolactone) are effective in treating HF in patients with HCM [26].

Beta blockers are the first drug of choice [1–3]. Progressively increasing the dosage of beta blockers in patients with rest obstruction is rarely effective in reducing gradient or symptoms, although it is possible to blunt exercise-provoked (labile) gradients [1–3]. Verapamil should be administered with caution to patients in advanced HF in the context of marked outflow obstruction [2, 3].

Disopyramide, a class Ia antiarrhythmic agent with potent negative inotropic properties, is an option for controlling HF symptoms in obstructive patients, and is the only drug shown to reduce rest gradient [27]. Its parasympathetic side effects have limited long-term efficacy, decreasing its widespread use [2, 3]. Although beneficial symptomatic responses are often achieved by the administration of cardioactive drugs to patients with HCM, conclusive evidence is lacking that pharmacological strategies can alter natural history or reduce mortality.

There is also no role for afterload reduction with angiotensin II receptor blockers (i.e., losartan), given that the prospective randomized INHERIT trial (INHibition of the renin angiotensin system in hypertrophic cardiomyopathy and the Effect on hypertrophy – a Randomized Intervention Trial with losartan) showed no change in the primary endpoint of LV mass reduction [28]. Now, for more than 30 years (since verapamil), no new drugs have been introduced to treat HF in HCM, representing an unmet need in this disease. Consequently, in HCM, non-pharmacological therapies have dominated the management of disabling HF symptoms.

SURGICAL SEPTAL MYECTOMY

Myectomy is the preferred ("gold standard") intervention for patients with HCM experiencing unacceptably impaired quality of life with exertional dyspnea which is refractory to maximum medical management (NYHA functional class III/IV), due to LV outflow obstruction (peak gradient ≥ 50 mm Hg at rest or with exercise), in accord with the American College of Cardiology/American Heart Association guidelines [2, 8].

Surgical myectomy benefits the clinical course in two major respects. First, surgery consistently abolishes subaortic gradient and impedance to LV outflow (and mitral regurgitation), in the process normalizing intracavity pressures [5, 29–31] by virtue of widening the outflow tract cross-sectional area and eliminating the drag effect on mitral valve and systolic anterior motion [32]. Based on the substantial data assembled from HCM centers worldwide over several decades, 90% to 95% of myectomy patients experience enhanced quality of life with no or only mild residual symptoms post-operatively [5, 29–31].

Second, gradient and symptom relief persist long term and are associated with a survival benefit equivalent to an age- and gender-matched general population, as well as a possibly reduced sudden death risk [5, 29–31]. The principle that HF symptoms in HCM are reversible with mechanical relief of outflow tract obstruction, restoring the vast majority of patients to a normal or near-normal lifestyle, is notable. Not only does this experience substantiate that outflow gradient is the predominant mechanism for exertional dyspnea, but clearly distinguishes HF in HCM from conventional congestive heart failure (CHF), which is associated with high morbidity and a mortality rate of 10% per year [33–35]. Indeed, even with current treatment initiatives, mortality from conventional CHF remains increased, while paradoxically mortality and morbidity in HCM are decreasing [24, 36].

Operative mortality has decreased from 6% (25 years ago) to only 0.4% (currently), when performed in experienced myectomy centers [37]. However, there is a relative paucity of surgeons experienced at myectomy, limiting access to this effective therapy for many patients [38]. Notably, HCM patients with HF due to physiologically provoked gradients also benefit from septal reduction similar to those with rest obstruction [16]. In a small proportion of cases (4%), myectomy fails to achieve symptom relief, even after abolition of gradient due to comorbidities and systolic or diastolic dysfunction [39].

ALCOHOL SEPTAL ABLATION

Percutaneous alcohol ablation, introduced 20 years ago, produces transmural basal septal infarction to relieve LV outflow gradient and HF symptoms [38, 39]. In accordance with the American College of Cardiology/American Heart Association guidelines, alcohol ablation is considered a therapeutic alternative to myectomy in selected patients, particularly those of advanced age or with comorbidities [2]. Although alcohol ablation can reduce obstruction and symptoms, the alcohol-induced septal scar can also create arrhythmogenic risk in susceptible patients [38].

Dual-chamber pacing, as an alternative to surgery, has been largely abandoned as ineffective, its benefits attributable to a placebo effect [40].

HEART TRANSPLANTATION

Treatment for advanced HF has acquired an increasingly prominent profile within the HCM disease spectrum, leading to transplantation as the only definitive treatment option in a minority of non-obstructive patients [4, 19, 20, 24]. Although patients with HCM with an EF of < 50% (and often LV remodeling) have been the traditional transplant candidates, notably about one-half of all severely symptomatic patients listed for transplant now show preserved systolic function (EF $\geq$ 50%).

Once progression to the end-stage and systolic dysfunction has occurred, pharmacological management includes angiotensin-converting enzyme inhibitors/angiotensin receptor blockers, betablockers, spironolactone, and digoxin. These drugs benefit patients with conventional CHF, but they have uncertain efficacy and do not reverse the clinical course or transplant recommendation in HCM [2, 3]. There are limited pharmacological options in this subgroup, similar in this respect to patients with preserved EF.

Transplantation occurs at a wide range of ages (16 to 66 years), but usually in mid-life (average 42 years) [19] with the time lapse between symptom onset and transplant listing averaging eight years, and between listing and transplantation only about six months [19]. These intervals underscore the importance of close longitudinal surveillance to monitor symptom progression [4, 19, 20, 24].

Notably, some young, severely limited patients with end-stage HCM may not be considered for transplant listing based on certain conventional criteria from the International Society for Heart and Lung Transplantation, namely, normal EF and/or peak myocardial oxygen consumption (VO_2) on CPET exceeding the recommended threshold (i.e., > 14 ml/kg/min or > 50% predicted for age) [22]. This VO_2 cutoff value for transplant listing is derived from experience with non-HCM cardiomyopathies and may not reliably reflect the daily symptom limitation experienced by patients with end-stage HCM [19]. This mismatch between peak VO_2 and exercise capacity can exclude some deserving severely symptomatic patients with HCM from heart transplant consideration, which is unfortunate since HCM patients have a post-transplant survival benefit similar to ischemic and other cardiomyopathies [41].

GENETICALLY BASED INTERVENTIONS

There have been therapies proposed to obliterate or prevent the overall HCM disease process, including pre-implantation genetic diagnosis and therapy. More recently, CRISPR-Cas9-based targeted gene editing has been used to correct inherited pathogenic gene mutations (e.g., MYBPC3 for HCM) in pre-implantation human embryos [42].

CONCLUSIONS

Hypertrophic cardiomyopathy is a contemporary treatable disease that has a worldwide prevalence. Despite this, treatment of this disease is challenged by lack of adequate resources, especially lack of experienced surgeons. The most distinctive characteristic of HCM is heart failure reversibility when mechanical impedance to LV outflow is relieved or abolished by surgical myectomy (or, selectively, alcohol septal ablation). In those patients at risk of SCD, ICD has shown mortality benefit. In the current management era for obstructive (as well as non-obstructive) HCM, there should be little reason for mortality attributable to HCM.

REFERENCES

1. B.J. Maron, S.R. Ommen, C. Semsarian, P. Spirito, I. Olivotto, M.S. Maron. Hypertrophic cardiomyopathy: present and future, with translation into contemporary cardiovascular medicine. *J Am Coll Cardiol*, 64 (2014), pp. 83–99
2. B.J. Gersh, B.J. Maron, R.O. Bonow, et al. ACCF/AHA guideline for the diagnosis and treatment of hypertrophic cardiomyopathy: executive summary: a report of the American College of Cardiology Foundation/American Heart Association Task Force on Practice Guidelines. *J Am Coll Cardiol*, 58 (2011), pp. 2703–2738
3. P.M. Elliott, A. Anastasakis, M.A. Borger, et al. ESC guidelines on diagnosis and management of hypertrophic cardiomyopathy. *Eur Heart J*, 35 (2014), pp. 2733–2779

4. D. Pasqualucci, A. Fornaro, G. Castelli, et al. Clinical spectrum, therapeutic options, and outcome of advanced heart failure in hypertrophic cardiomyopathy. *Circ Heart Fail*, 8 (2015), pp. 1014–1021

5. S.R. Ommen, B.J. Maron, I. Olivotto, et al. Long-term effects of surgical septal myectomy on survival in patients with obstructive hypertrophic cardiomyopathy. *J Am Coll Cardiol*, 46 (2005), pp. 470–476

6. M.V. Sherrid, S. Balaram, B. Kim, L. Axel, D.G. Swistel. The mitral valve in obstructive hypertrophic cardiomyopathy: a test in context. *J Am Coll Cardiol*, 67 (2016), pp. 1846–1858

7. E.J. Rowin, B.J. Maron, T.S. Haas, et al. Hypertrophic cardiomyopathy with left ventricular apical aneurysm: implications for risk stratification and management. *J Am Coll Cardiol*, 69 (2017), pp. 761–773

8. M.S. Maron, I. Olivotto, S. Betocchi, et al. Effect of left ventricular outflow tract obstruction on clinical outcome in hypertrophic cardiomyopathy. *N Engl J Med*, 348 (2003), pp. 295–303

9. B.J. Maron, E.J. Rowin, S.A. Casey, et al. Risk stratification and outcome of patients with hypertrophic cardiomyopathy ≥ 60 years of age. *Circulation*, 127 (2013), pp. 585–593

10. E. Biagini, P. Spirito, G. Rocchi, et al. Prognostic implications of the Doppler restrictive filling pattern in hypertrophic cardiomyopathy. *Am J Cardiol*, 104 (2009), pp. 1727–1731

11. F. Cecchi, I. Olivotto, R. Gistri, R. Lorenzoni, G. Chiriatti, P.G. Camici. Coronary microvascular dysfunction and prognosis in hypertrophic cardiomyopathy. *N Engl J Med*, 349 (2003), pp. 1027–1035

12. C.J. Coats, K. Rantell, A. Bartnik, et al. Cardiopulmonary exercise testing and prognosis in hypertrophic cardiomyopathy. *Circ Heart Fail*, 8 (2015), pp. 1022–1031

13. A. Masri, L.M. Pierson, N.G. Smedira, et al. Predictors of long-term outcomes in patients with hypertrophic cardiomyopathy undergoing cardiopulmonary stress testing and echocardiography. *Am Heart J*, 169 (2015), pp. 684–692.e1

14. M. Covella, E.J. Rowin, N.S. Hill, et al. Mechanism of progressive heart failure and significance of pulmonary hypertension in obstructive hypertrophic cardiomyopathy. *Circ Heart Fail*, 10 (2017), Article e003689

15. J.B. Geske, T. Konecny, S.R. Ommen, et al. Surgical myectomy improves pulmonary hypertension in obstructive hypertrophic cardiomyopathy. *Eur Heart J*, 35 (2014), pp. 2032–2039

16. M.S. Maron, I. Olivotto, A.G. Zenovich, et al. Hypertrophic cardiomyopathy is predominantly a disease of left ventricular outflow tract obstruction. *Circulation*, 114 (2006), pp. 2232–2239

17. V.V. Le, M.V. Perez, M.T. Wheeler, J. Myers, I. Schnittger, E.A. Ashley. Mechanisms of exercise intolerance in patients with hypertrophic cardiomyopathy. *Am Heart J*, 158 (2009), pp. e27–e34

18. M.S. Maron, E.J. Rowin, I. Olivotto, et al. Contemporary natural history and management of nonobstructive hypertrophic cardiomyopathy. *J Am Coll Cardiol*, 67 (2016), pp. 1399–1409

19. E.J. Rowin, B.J. Maron, M.S. Kiernan, et al. Advanced heart failure with preserved systolic function in nonobstructive hypertrophic cardiomyopathy: under-recognized subset of candidates for heart transplant. *Circ Heart Fail*, 7 (2014), pp. 967–975

20. K.M. Harris, P. Spirito, M.S. Maron, et al. Prevalence, clinical profile, and significance of left ventricular remodeling in the end-stage phase of hypertrophic cardiomyopathy. *Circulation*, 114 (2006), pp. 216–225

21. P. Sorajja, T. Allison, C. Hayes, R.A. Nishimura, C.S. Lam, S.R. Ommen. Prognostic utility of metabolic exercise testing in minimally symptomatic patients with obstructive hypertrophic cardiomyopathy. *Am J Cardiol*, 109 (2012), pp. 1494–1498

22. M.R. Mehra, J. Kobashigawa, R. Starling, et al. Listing criteria for heart transplantation: International Society for Heart and Lung Transplantation guidelines for the care of cardiac transplant candidates–2006. *J Heart Lung Transplant*, 25 (2006), pp. 1024–1042

23. J.B. Geske, P.M. McKie, S.R. Ommen, P. Sorajja. B-type natriuretic peptide and survival in hypertrophic cardiomyopathy. *J Am Coll Cardiol*, 61 (2013), pp. 2456–2460

24. B.J. Maron, E.J. Rowin, S.A. Casey, M.S. Maron. How hypertrophic cardiomyopathy became a contemporary treatable genetic disease with low mortality. *JAMA Cardiol.*, 1 (2016), p. 98

25. D.M. Gilligan, W.L. Chan, J. Joshi, et al. A double-blind, placebo-controlled crossover trial of nadolol and verapamil in mild and moderately symptomatic hypertrophic cardiomyopathy. *J Am Coll Cardiol*, 21 (1993), pp. 1672–1679

26. M.S. Maron, R.H. Chan, N. Kapur, et al. Effect of spironolactone on myocardial fibrosis and other clinical variables in patients with hypertrophic cardiomyopathy: a prospective, randomized trial. Paper presented at: *American Heart Association Scientific Sessions*; November 16–20, 2013; Dallas, TX

27. M.V. Sherrid, I. Barac, W.J. McKenna, et al. Multicenter study of the efficacy and safety of disopyramide in obstructive hypertrophic cardiomyopathy. *J Am Coll Cardiol*, 45 (2005), pp. 1251–1258

28. A. Axelsson, K. Iversen, N. Vejlstrup, et al. Efficacy and safety of the angiotensin II receptor blocker losartan for hypertrophic cardiomyopathy. *Lancet Diab Endocrinol*, 3 (2015), pp. 123–131

29. A. Woo, W.G. Williams, R. Choi, et al. Clinical and echocardiographic determinants of long-term survival after surgical myectomy in obstructive hypertrophic cardiomyopathy. *Circulation*, 111 (2005), pp. 2033–2041

30. M.Y. Desai, A. Bhonsale, N.G. Smedira, et al. Predictors of long-term outcomes in symptomatic hypertrophic obstructive cardiomyopathy patients undergoing surgical relief of left ventricular outflow tract obstruction. *Circulation*, 128 (2013), pp. 209–216

31. H. Rastegar, G. Boll, E.J. Rowin, et al. Results of surgical septal myectomy for obstructive hypertrophic cardiomyopathy: the Tufts experience. *Ann Cardiothorac Surg*, 6 (2017), pp. 353–363

32. P. Spirito, B.J. Maron, D.R. Rosing. Morphologic determinants of hemodynamic state after ventricular septal myotomy-myectomy in patients with obstructive hypertrophic cardiomyopathy: M mode and two-dimensional echocardiographic assessment. *Circulation*, 70 (1984), pp. 984–995

33. E. Braunwald. The war against heart failure: the Lancet lecture. *Lancet*, 385 (2015), pp. 812–824

34. P. Ponikowski, A.A. Voors, S.D. Anker, et al. 2016 ESC Guidelines for the diagnosis and treatment of acute and chronic heart failure. *Eur Heart J*, 37 (2016), pp. 2129–2200

35. C.W. Yancy, M. Jessup, B. Bozkurt, et al. 2017 ACC/AHA/HFSA focused Update of the 2013 ACCF/AHA Guideline for the Management of Heart Failure. *J Am Coll Cardiol*, 70 (2017), pp. 776–779

36. B.J. Maron, E.J. Rowin, S.A. Casey, et al. Hypertrophic cardiomyopathy in adulthood associated with low cardiovascular mortality with contemporary management strategies. *J Am Coll Cardiol*, 65 (2015), pp. 1915–1928

37. B.J. Maron, J.A. Dearani, S.R. Ommen, et al. Low operative mortality achieved with surgical septal myectomy: role of dedicated hypertrophic cardiomyopathy centers in the management of dynamic subaortic obstruction. *J Am Coll Cardiol*, 66 (2015), pp. 1307–1308

38. B.J. Maron, R.A. Nishimura. Surgical septal myectomy versus alcohol septal ablation: assessing the status of the controversy in 2014. *Circulation*, 130 (2014), pp. 1617–1624

39. P. Sorajja, S.R. Ommen, D.R. Holmes Jr., et al. Survival after alcohol septal ablation for obstructive hypertrophic cardiomyopathy. *Circulation*, 126 (2012), pp. 2374–2380

40. B.J. Maron, R.A. Nishimura, W.J. McKenna, H. Rakowski, M.E. Josephson, R.S. Kieval. Assessment of permanent dual-chamber pacing as a treatment for drug-refractory symptomatic patients with obstructive hypertrophic cardiomyopathy. A randomized, double-blind, crossover study (M-PATHY). *Circulation*, 99 (1999), pp. 2927–2933

41. A.M. Killu, J.Y. Park, J.D. Sara, et al. Cardiac resynchronization therapy in patients with end-stage hypertrophic cardiomyopathy. *Europace*, 20 (2018), pp. 82–88

42. H. Ma, N. Marti-Gutierrez, S.-W. Park, et al. Correction of a pathogenic gene mutation in human embryos. *Nature*, 548 (2017), pp. 413–419

Chapter 2

GENETICS AND GENETIC TESTING IN HYPERTROPHIC CARDIOMYOPATHY

Hashim Ahamed

CONTENTS

INTRODUCTION

Hypertrophic cardiomyopathy (HCM) is a common inherited heart disease with a prevalence of at least 1:500 [1–8]. It is defined by the presence of left ventricular hypertrophy (LVH) in the absence of causal cardiac or systemic disease. It can lead to significant cardiovascular morbidity and mortality, including heart failure and sudden cardiac death (SCD). The world over, it is the commonest cause of SCD in the young. Hypertrophic cardiomyopathy is classically regarded as an autosomal dominant Mendelian disease, with variable expressivity and penetrance. More than one thousand variants in eight sarcomeric genes have since been linked to HCM and almost 250 variants in over 40 additional, mainly non-sarcomeric, genes have also been implicated in HCM, mostly identified through candidate gene research studies involving genes with a hypothetical role. It is becoming increasingly clear that an accurate genetic characterization and thorough phenotyping of these patients is the key to understanding the disease process and ultimately leading to improved patient outcomes and effective family screening strategies.

Hypertrophic cardiomyopathy phenocopies are disease processes which resemble HCM in phenotypic characteristics, but are distinct entities which can only be distinguished by their unique genotypic profile. It is critical to make this distinction to prevent catastrophic consequences of mischaracterization, a distinction which can only be performed with next-generation genetic analysis and deep phenotyping.

GENETICS OF HCM

Hypertrophic cardiomyopathy is caused by dominant mutations in 11 or more genes which encode thick and thin contractile myofilament protein components of the sarcomere or the adjacent Z-disk (Figures 2.1 and 2.3) [9–12]. Seventy percent of the mutations are in two genes – the β-myosin heavy chain (MYH7) and the myosin-binding protein C (MYBPC3). To underscore the vast genetic heterogeneity of HCM, over the past 20 years more than 1,400 mutations (largely missense) have been identified [8, 9]. Pathogenic mutations that cause HCM are transmitted in an autosomal dominant pattern; every offspring of an affected relative has a 50% chance of inheritance and risk of developing disease [9–13], although sporadic cases do arise due to *de novo* mutations. Phenotypic heterogeneity is evident between and within families, suggesting that mutations of the sarcomere are not the sole determinant of the HCM phenotype. Age-related penetrance may result in the delayed appearance of LVH in the third decade and beyond [14, 15]. Therefore, HCM can be considered as one heterogeneous disease entity rather than a conglomeration of similar but unrelated disorders [12–15].

GENETIC TESTING IN HCM

Genetic testing is now more frequently offered in dedicated HCM clinics according to established professional guidelines [16–18]. The knowledge thus revealed through genetic testing has considerable implications for the index patient with HCM and other members in the family. The genetic information can thus identify relatives in the family with clinically unrecognized HCM, individuals who are at risk of developing the condition, and other members of the family who do not carry the pathogenic mutation, who do not need further periodic clinical screening. Therefore, it is of paramount importance that a center of excellence for HCM should have dedicated personnel who understand the basic tenets of genetic testing in the condition and who are thus a core component of the multidisciplinary team [19].

THE ROLE OF GENETIC COUNSELING IN HCM GENETIC TESTING SERVICES

Genetic counselors play an invaluable role in the management of a patient with HCM and their families by providing important perspectives regarding the testing process and the subsequent genetic information that it may reveal. Their role is defined by:

1   Eliciting a detailed family history;
2   Educating regarding the principles of genetic disease and its implications;
3   Helping the patient and family to understand the types of genetic testing and offering psychological support;
4   Translating the results of genetic testing to the patient and family, in order to help them make informed choices (e.g., reproductive implications);
5   Coordinating the process of informed consent prior to genetic testing and communicating the advantages and limitations of each type of test.

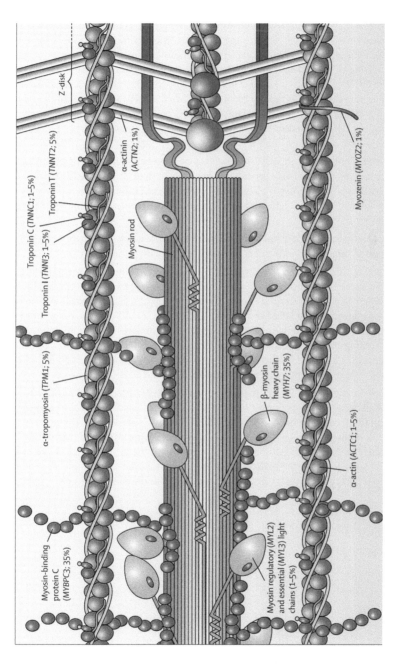

Figure 2.1 HCM is caused by dominant mutations in 11 or more genes encoding thick and thin contractile myofilament protein components of the sarcomere or the adjacent Z-disk.

The utility of clinical genetic testing can be understood by dividing it into the following two broad categories.

Diagnostic testing. This is performed to identify the underlying genetic etiology in a patient with established or suspected HCM, yielding a specific, etiology-based diagnosis. In clinical situations where the crude clinical phenotype of HCM mimics other conditions (phenocopies), this form of testing will be able to establish the diagnosis of sarcomeric HCM and thus differentiate it from HCM phenocopies. For example, conditions like Fabry disease and cardiac amyloidosis may mimic the phenotype of sarcomeric HCM. These HCM mimics can be reliably differentiated from sarcomeric HCM by genetic testing. It is imperative to establish this distinction since the HCM phenocopies have entirely different management strategies and prognosis.

Apart from establishing a genetic diagnosis, recent evidence seems to indicate that the presence of certain sarcomeric variants may predict adverse clinical outcomes in HCM patients. The clinical implication of this genotype–phenotype correlation is an evolving one, and larger studies need to be done to validate a genetic variant-guided management strategy in HCM patients and their families.

Once a pathogenic genetic variant has been identified in a patient, this information can be used to pursue targeted cascade screening of at-risk individuals in the patient's family.

Predictive testing. The inheritance pattern of HCM is autosomal dominant, which means that there is a 50% chance of transmission to each offspring. In this context, the evaluation of at-risk family members is important. The aim of performing predictive testing in a family is to identify individuals with unrecognized HCM and individuals who are at risk and who will benefit from longitudinal cardiovascular follow-up. For individuals at risk of developing HCM, longitudinal follow-up screening consists of ECG and an echocardiogram, which is repeated every one to five years, depending on age and other risk factors in the family. An example of predictive testing in a family with an HCM proband is shown in Figure 2.2.

If a relative of a patient with HCM (with a pathogenic DNA variant) tests positive for the same variant as the proband, then that individual is at risk of developing HCM and should continue with the recommended longitudinal cardiovascular surveillance. If a relative tests negative for the pathogenic DNA variant, then that individual can be offered reassurance that they are unlikely to develop HCM or transmit the disease to the next generation and can be potentially released from a systematic longitudinal cardiovascular screening with a recommendation to report to clinical services if there is a change in the clinical status. Even though

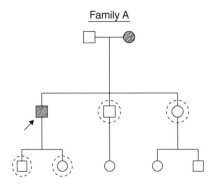

Figure 2.2 An example of predictive testing in a family with an HCM proband.

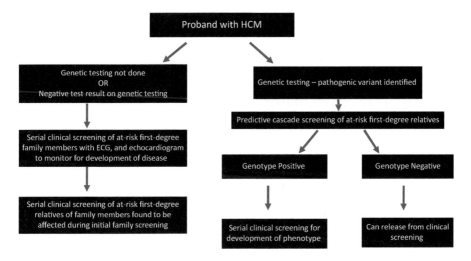

Figure 2.3   The various pathways of predictive genetic testing in HCM patients.

an at-risk member of the family tests negative for the pathogenic variant identified in a relative with HCM, a baseline cardiac clinical evaluation (electrocardiogram and echocardiogram) is always recommended. The various pathways of predictive genetic testing in HCM patients is shown in Figure 2.3.

There are certain factors which will determine the pre-test probability that genetic testing in HCM will yield clinically valuable information. These factors must always be taken into account when counseling HCM patients for genetic testing and they include:

1   Familial pattern of inheritance: A familial disease will increase the pre-test probability of identifying a pathogenic variant in more than 50% of cases.

2   Patients with atypical HCM morphology or with a clinical background that can trigger LVH, such as athletic conditioning or systemic hypertension, are less likely to have a pathogenic HCM variant identified.

3   If there are other family members who have established HCM in addition to the patient being tested, then this adds value to the genetic testing as segregation analysis may be carried out to determine the significance of the isolated DNA variant.

In summary, the following are the clinical scenarios which would influence the utility of genetic testing in HCM:

1   Genetic testing is high yield: There is presence of typical HCM morphology on cardiac imaging and a familial pattern of disease.

2   Genetic testing is intermediate yield: Atypical HCM morphology on cardiac imaging and relatives with established HCM are available for segregation analysis.

3   Genetic testing is low yield: HCM morphology is poorly defined and there are no relatives with established HCM and no evidence of a familial pattern of inheritance.

GENETIC TESTING IN HCM: SEQUENTIAL STEPS

STEP 1: DEFINE THE APPROPRIATE PATIENT TO TEST

Building a multi-generation family pedigree is important to delineate family relationships and the presence of significant medical history. This will identify the presence of familial disease and the ideal proband to be subjected to testing. The person to be tested in the family should ideally be the individual with the most severe form of HCM, which in turn is determined by clinical presentation, cardiac imaging, and adverse clinical outcomes. The family pedigree analysis will also highlight the presence of at-risk members who will qualify for predictive cascade genetic testing.

STEP 2: CHOOSE THE APPROPRIATE GENETIC TEST

Multi-gene panels are commonly used for HCM genetic testing. Different laboratories, commercial or research based, will have variations in the composition of their gene panels. But, generally, the panels will often include a wide array of sarcomere genes, which have a proven genetic basis with the phenotypic expression of HCM. An HCM genetic panel will usually include well-described sarcomere genes such as myosin-binding protein C (MYBPC3), the myosin heavy chain (MYH7), cardiac troponin T(TNNT2), cardiac troponin I (TNNI3), alpha-tropomyosin (TPM1), myosin essential and regulatory light chains (MYL2, MYL3), and cardiac actin (ACTC) [8].

An important point to note while performing HCM genetic testing concerns HCM phenocopies. These entities may mimic the phenotypic expression of sarcomeric HCM. Fabry disease, Danon disease, Pompe disease, and mitochondrial myopathy syndromes often have cardiac and extracardiac manifestations which may serve as red flags, thus prompting the genetic testing for these diseases. Therefore, it is clinically important to ensure that the common HCM phenocopies are also included in the HCM genetic panel, as the diagnosis of these phenocopies will allow for unique risk stratification and management strategies, which are different as compared to sarcomeric HCM.

Of late, the HCM genetic testing strategy has seen an expansion in terms of the type of testing pursued. Whole exome sequencing and whole genome sequencing are more comprehensive than gene panels and have been utilized as a genetic testing strategy in many HCM centers. However, similar to the data obtained from using large HCM gene panels, it is also becoming evident that using more broader testing strategies like whole exome sequencing or whole genome sequencing may not significantly improve the detection rates for a pathogenic variant related to HCM. The disadvantage of broader testing strategies is that they increase the possibility of detecting incidental genetic variants which may be unrelated to HCM (e.g., cancer related), thus genetic counseling strategies must be in place to discuss the potential psychological harm that this may entail. However, it does appear that broad genetic testing services will be increasingly utilized in the future.

STEP 3: PRE-TEST COUNSELING AND INFORMED CONSENT

As discussed in the section on the role of genetic counseling in HCM genetic testing, pre-test counseling along with informed consent are core elements of the testing process. This will enable the patient to understand the important principles of the testing process and practical implications of the genetic test results. This is a critical step for the patient, as this allows the individual to make an informed decision about whether to undergo genetic testing or not. The genetic counselor will be able to prime the patient and their families regarding the possible psychological or social sequelae that may arise from such a testing process.

STEP 4: REVIEW AND INTERPRETATION OF GENETIC TEST REPORTS

The process of genetic testing in HCM will finally lead to the identification of certain DNA variants. The most critical step, now, is to determine whether the variant identified is the cause of HCM in the given patient. In other words, the testing process now has to assess the pathogenicity of the identified variant or variants. This process of determining pathogenicity is an imperfect science due to the complexity of the human genome. In addition, there may be a distinct lack of functional studies pertaining to the variant identified, which, if present, would have demonstrated that the variant has a physiological effect on the cardiovascular system.

The report generated by the testing laboratory will classify the variant identified based on their assessment of the probability that it is the cause of HCM in a given patient. This reporting framework is based on guidelines issued by the American College of Medical Genetics and Genomics (ACMG) and the Association for Molecular Pathology. There are various tools in the public domain, such as Gnomad [20], Clinvar [21], Exac [20], and ClinGen [22], which can aid the interpretation process of the variants identified by genetic testing. The genetic testing laboratory classifies variants as follows.

1 Benign variant;

2 Likely benign variant;

3 Variant of uncertain significance (VUS);

4 Likely pathogenic variant;

5 Pathogenic variant.

A positive genetic test would involve the identification of pathogenic or likely pathogenic variants. The identification of a pathogenic variant in HCM genetic testing will provide a genetic basis for the phenotypic manifestation of HCM in a given patient. This pathogenic variant can be used to perform predictive cascade testing in other at-risk members of the family. The value of a likely pathogenic variant is less certain in terms of its ability to cause the disease in an individual. Caution must be exercised in using likely pathogenic variants for cascade screening in the family.

Variants of uncertain significance do not provide a genetic basis for HCM. As a result, VUSs cannot be used for predictive cascade testing in the family. However, if an additional family member with established HCM also carries the same variant (which had been identified as a VUS in the proband), then the variant may be considered a reliable marker of HCM within that particular family (since the VUS is co-segregated with the phenotype). Whenever a VUS is identified, the greater the number of relatives are found to be affected with HCM and have the same VUS as the proband, the more likely that the identified VUS is the cause of HCM in that particular family. This segregation analysis is an important process for further clarification regarding the pathogenicity of a VUS.

A likely benign or benign-variant result is considered to be a negative test result when the reports are interpreted. However, since the diagnostic yield of genetic testing is between 40 and 60%, a negative genetic test result does not exclude the absence of a genetic basis for HCM in a given patient. If the initial testing strategy was a genetic panel, a broader testing strategy may be pursued in these patients with an initial negative test result. Family clinical screening is still recommended in these patients.

VARIANT CLASSIFICATION: A DYNAMIC PROCESS

Classification of a variant by a laboratory is based on the accumulated evidence at that point in time. The initial classification may change over time as new evidence for a particular variant emerges [23, 24]. If a variant is reclassified, it is imperative that the patient and the family are contacted again, and any changes in testing or management strategy must be communicated. If a pathogenic variant is reclassified as a VUS, family members who were initially released from longitudinal screening may have to be asked to continue periodic clinical evaluation. If a VUS is reclassified as pathogenic, then additional testing strategies like predictive cascade screening needs to be offered to the family along with periodic clinical screening.

SPECIAL CONSIDERATIONS: HCM PHENOCOPIES

Certain myocardial storage cardiomyopathies may mimic the phenotypic manifestations of sarcomeric HCM and they are an important differential diagnosis in the work-up of a patient with the HCM phenotype. They include:

1   Danon disease, an X-linked dominant lyosomal storage disorder;

2   Fabry disease, an X-linked recessive disease due to mutations in the galactosidase alpha (GLA) geneand α-galactosidase A deficiency leading to multiorgan intracellular glycosphingolipid deposition;

3   PRKAG 2 disease, with mutations in the regulatory subunit of adenosine monophosphate-activated protein kinase.

These entities account for approximately < 1% of those patients presenting with a clinical diagnosis of HCM [25–29]. Application of genetic testing in these phenocopies, which may have been initially misdiagnosed clinically, will lead to an appropriate genetic and disease-specific diagnosis. This is of critical importance, as these mimics of HCM have an entirely different natural history, risk stratification protocols, and management modalities.

For example, Danon disease is associated with a rapidly progressive clinical course with a high frequency of lethal arrhythmias within the first three decades of life; these patients require an early referral for cardiac transplantation [26, 27]. Similarly, in Fabry disease, early institution of enzyme replacement therapy in the form of recombinant alpha-galactosidase A may potentially lead to regression of LVH and improvement in various cardiovascular performance indicators [28, 29].

The pre-test probability of detecting these HCM phenocopies is governed by the presence of certain clinical red flags encountered during the work-up of these patients. These red flags may include Wolff–Parkinson–White pattern in PRKAG2 and Danon disease, greatly increased precordial voltages, and massive LVH in patients with LAMP2 mutations (Danon disease) [25, 27] and symmetric LVH with late gadolinium enhancement of the posterobasal LV seen in Fabry disease [28, 29].

HYPERTROPHIC CARDIOMYOPATHY GENETIC TESTING IN INDIA: LOGISTICS

Genetic testing for HCM in India has become more accessible in the last decade. The costs associated with a genetic panel or a clinical exome have consistently fallen over the years and genetic testing in these patients has now become a practical mode of investigation. The sample of choice for genetic testing is peripheral blood, although other sources of DNA such as buccal swab, dried blood spot, and saliva are viable options.

CONCLUSION

Genetic testing is a potent tool in the investigation and management of patients with HCM and identification of at-risk healthy family members. It is becoming increasingly available now, and it is important that the practicing cardiologists familiarize themselves with the advantages, limitations, and nuances which underline the complexities of genetic testing. When genetic testing is integrated into the clinical workflow of HCM patients, it adds the dimension of personalized medicine to the multidisciplinary management of HCM patients.

REFERENCES

1. Braunwald E, Lambrew CT, Rockoff SD, Ross J Jr, Morrow AG. Idiopathic hypertrophic subaortic stenosis, I: a description of the disease based upon an analysis of 64 patients. *Circulation* 1964;30:3–119.
2. Wigle ED, Rakowski H, Kimball BP, Williams WG. Hypertrophic cardiomyopathy: clinical spectrum and treatment. *Circulation* 1995;92:1680–1692.
3. Maron BJ. Hypertrophic cardiomyopathy: an important global disease. *Am J Med* 2004;116:63–65.
4. Maron BJ. Hypertrophic cardiomyopathy: a systematic review. *JAMA* 2002;287:1308–1320.
5. Alcalai R, Seidman JG, Seidman CE. Genetic basis of hypertrophic cardiomyopathy: from bench to the clinics. *J Cardiovasc Electrophysiol* 2008;19:104–110.
6. Maron BJ. Contemporary insights and strategies for risk stratification and prevention of sudden death in hypertrophic cardiomyopathy. *Circulation* 2010;121:445–456.
7. Maron BJ, McKenna WJ, Danielson GK, et al., and the Task Force on Clinical Expert Consensus Documents. A report of the American College of Cardiology Foundation Task Force on Clinical Expert Consensus Documents and the European Society of Cardiology Committee for Practice Guidelines. *J Am Coll Cardiol* 2003;42:1687–1713.
8. Seidman CE, Seidman JG. Identifying sarcomere gene mutations in hypertrophic cardiomyopathy: a personal history. *Circ Res* 2011;108:743–750.
9. Ackerman MJ, Van Driest SL, Ommen SR, et al. Prevalence and age-dependence of malignant mutations in the beta-myosin heavy chain and troponin T genes in hypertrophic cardiomyopathy: a comprehensive outpatient perspective. *J Am Coll Cardiol* 2002;39:2042–2048.
10. Niimura H, Bachinski LL, Sangwatanaroj S, et al. Mutations in the gene for cardiac myosin-binding protein C and late-onset familial hypertrophic cardiomyopathy. *N Engl J Med* 1998;338:1248–1257.
11. Van Driest SL, Ackerman MJ, Ommen SR, et al. Prevalence and severity of "benign" mutations in the beta-myosin heavy chain, cardiactroponin T, and alpha-tropomyosin genes in hypertrophic cardiomyopathy. *Circulation* 2002;106:3085–3090.
12. Landstrom AP, Ackerman MJ. Mutation type is not clinically useful in predicting prognosis in hypertrophic cardiomyopathy. *Circulation* 2010;122:2441–2449.
13. Richard P, Charron P, Carrier L, et al., and the EUROGENE Heart Failure Project. Hypertrophic cardiomyopathy: distribution of disease genes, spectrum of mutations, and implications for a molecular diagnosis strategy. *Circulation* 2003;107:2227–2232.
14. Ho CY. Genetics and clinical destiny: improving care in hypertrophic cardiomyopathy. *Circulation* 2010;122:2430–2440.
15. Maron BJ, Casey SA, Poliac LC, Gohman TE, Almquist AK, Aeppli DM. Clinical course of hypertrophic cardiomyopathy in a regional United States cohort. *JAMA* 1999;281:650–655.
16. Gersh BJ, Maron BJ, Bonow RO, et al. 2011 ACCF/AHA guideline for the diagnosis and treatment of hypertrophic cardiomyopathy: a report of the American College of Cardiology Foundation/American Heart Association Task Force on Practice Guidelines. *Circulation* 2011;124(24):e783–e831.
17. Hershberger RE, Givertz MM, Ho CY, et al. Genetic evaluation of cardiomyopathy – a Heart Failure Society of America practice guideline. *J Card Fail* 2018;24(5):281–302.
18. Elliott PM, Anastasakis A, Borger MA, et al. 2014 ESC guidelines on diagnosis and management of hypertrophic cardiomyopathy: the task force for the diagnosis and management of hypertrophic cardiomyopathy of the European Society of Cardiology (ESC). *Eur Heart J* 2014;35(39):2733–2779.
19. van Velzen HG, Schinkel AFL, Baart SJ, et al. Outcomes of contemporary family screening in hypertrophic cardiomyopathy. *Circ Genom Precis Med* 2018;11(4):e001896.

20. Lek M, Karczewski KJ, Minikel EV, et al. Analysis of protein-coding genetic variation in 60,706 humans. *Nature* 2016;536(7616):285–291.
21. Harrison SM, Riggs ER, Maglott DR, et al. Using ClinVar as a resource to support variant interpretation. *Curr Protoc Hum Genet* 2016;89:8.16.1–8.16.23.
22. Rehm HL, Berg JS, Brooks LD, et al. ClinGen – the clinical genome resource. *N Engl J Med* 2015;372(23):2235–2242.
23. Das KJ, Ingles J, Bagnall RD, et al. Determining pathogenicity of genetic variants in hypertrophic cardiomyopathy: importance of periodic reassessment. *Genet Med* 2014;16(4):286–293.
24. Walsh R, Thomson K, Ware JS, et al. Reassessment of Mendelian gene pathogenicity using 7,855 cardiomyopathy cases and 60,706 reference samples. *Genet Med* 2017;19(2):192–203.
25. Arad M, Maron BJ, Gorham JM, et al. Glycogen storage diseases presenting as hypertrophic cardiomyopathy. *N Engl J Med* 2005;352:362–372.
26. Maron BJ, Roberts WC, Arad M, et al. Clinical outcome and phenotypic expression in LAMP2 cardiomyopathy. *JAMA* 2009;301:1253–1259.
27. Maron BJ, Ho CY, Kitner C, et al. Profound left ventricular remodeling associated with LAMP2 cardiomyopathy. *Am J Cardiol* 2010;106:1194–1196.
28. Weidemann F, Niemann M, Breunig F, et al. Long-term effects of enzyme replacement therapy on Fabry cardiomyopathy: evidence for a better outcome with early treatment. *Circulation* 2009;119:524–529.
29. Patel MR, Cecchi F, Cizmarik M, et al. Cardiovascular events in patients with Fabry disease: Natural history data from the Fabry registry. *J Am Coll Cardiol* 2011;57:1093–1099.

Chapter 3

NATURAL HISTORY OF HYPERTROPHIC CARDIOMYOPATHY

Srilakshmi M. Adhyapak

CONTENTS

INTRODUCTION

Hypertrophic cardiomyopathy (HCM) is a disease entity characterized by marked heterogeneity in morphology and natural history. Patients range in age from infants [1] to the elderly [2], and the clinical spectrum varies from the asymptomatic form to sudden death as an initial presentation. Most data on the natural history of the disease has been obtained from tertiary hospital referrals.

THE NATURAL HISTORY OF HCM IN CHILDREN FROM TERTIARY HOSPITAL DATA

The progression of left ventricular hypertrophy over three to six years has been identified in > 70% of children with HCM [3]. In many the progression of hypertrophy was striking, with increases in wall thickness of more than 20 mm (250%). This progression was noticed as not being associated with clinical deterioration, and most of the children remained symptom free.

Remodeling of left ventricular morphology and geometry during childhood can also lead to changes in the hemodynamics of the disease. Children, in whom the increase in wall thickness leads to a substantial decrease in the size of the left ventricular outflow tract so as to cause an anterior displacement of the mitral valve, develop systolic anterior motion of the mitral leaflets and dynamic obstruction to outflow [4]. While progression of left ventricular hypertrophy is common in children, especially during adolescence, it has not been identified in adults [5]. The fact that progression of hypertrophy is confined to a period of rapid body growth suggests that the factors that are responsible for growth and development during childhood may have an important role in this increase in left ventricular wall thickness.

In adults, left ventricular remodeling results from progressive left ventricular wall thinning and cavity dilatation. These changes in wall thickness are also associated with a progressive increase in left ventricular cavity dimension, though absolute left ventricular dilatation is rare. Marked wall thinning, relative cavity dilatation, and systolic dysfunction have been reported in about 10% of patients with HCM and moderate-to-severe symptoms [6]. Therefore, this malignant morphological evolution with extensive left ventricular remodeling occurs in a significant minority of patients with symptoms. At necropsy, the hearts of patients with wall thinning and cavity dilatation show diffuse left ventricular scarring, usually of both the septum and the left ventricular free wall. The mechanisms responsible for myocardial scarring and wall thinning in HCM have not been established. It is likely, however, that chronic ischemia plays an important part in scarring. Several studies have shown myocardial ischemia in HCM [7–9]. Ischemia could be caused by inadequate capillary density relative to the increased myocardial mass. In addition, abnormal intramyocardial arterioles with thickened walls and an apparently narrowed lumen have been described in HCM [10] and may contribute to myocardial ischemia.

The clinical course and natural history of HCM is the result of a complex interaction of left ventricular hypertrophy, left ventricular remodeling, and several functional alterations, including diastolic impairment, myocardial ischemia, outflow tract obstruction, and arrhythmias.

Because the severity of each of these morphological and functional abnormalities varies greatly across patients, the clinical course and natural history of the disease are extremely heterogeneous. In some patients symptoms never develop, in some severe symptoms of heart failure develop, and others die suddenly and unexpectedly, often in the absence of previous cardiac symptoms [11–13]. There is indirect evidence, however, that many patients have a more benign clinical course than could be inferred from most published reports. This conclusion is based on several points. Most patients with severe symptoms are referred to a few selected tertiary centers and the majority of the data published on HCM has come from these referral institutions and constitute, in large measure, what we know about HCM. Because these referral centers see the most critically ill patients and publish many studies on HCM, it is likely that the image of the disease that is projected into published reports is worse than the "real disease" in the overall patient population. This conclusion was also supported by the results of genetic studies performed on large numbers of families with HCM. In a study in which almost 300 relatives of patients with HCM were systematically investigated, a quarter of the relatives were found to be affected [14]. More than 70% of these relatives were symptom free. Studies based on patients from non-referral centers reported mortality for HCM that was substantially lower than the generally quoted figures of 3–4% a year [15–17].

PROGNOSTIC FACTORS FOR SURVIVAL

The factors influencing survival in HCM were obtained from a meta-analysis of pooled data from 13 studies [18]. Here average age, NYHA functional class, non-sustained ventricular tachycardia, family history of sudden death, syncope, atrial fibrillation, maximum left ventricular wall thickness, and obstruction either in the outflow tract or mid-ventricular region were significant prognostic factors for cardiovascular death. Conversely, for all-cause death, average age and family history of sudden cardiac death were not significant prognostic factors. For sudden cardiac death, non-sustained ventricular tachycardia, family history of sudden cardiac death, and obstruction were significantly predictive. Furthermore, NYHA class III/IV was the most important risk factor for cardiovascular death (HR = 2.53, 95% CI [2.10, 3.07]); maximum left ventricular wall thickness was the most important risk factor for sudden cardiac death (HR = 3.17, 95% CI [1.64, 6.12]); whereas NYHA class III/IV showed the strongest prognostic value for all-cause death (HR = 1.96, 95% CI [1.58, 2.43]).

In another study on the natural history of non-obstructive HCM, a cohort of 600 patients was followed over 24 months [19]. All patients were in NYHA class I/II. Only 10% of patients progressed to NYHA class III/IV. These patients were deemed to be transplant candidates. The risk factors for progression to worsening heart failure were many. They were more likely to be symptomatic at the baseline in class II (62% vs. 24%; p < 0.001), also to have larger left atria (46 ± 8 mm vs. 39 ±7 mm; p < 0.001), a more frequent history of atrial fibrillation (58% vs. 15%; p < 0.001), lower ejection fraction (EF) (60 ± 8% vs. 63 ± 6%; p = 0.04), and more extensive late gadolinium enhancement (LGE) (15 ± 14% vs. 6 ± 9%; p = 0.008). With multivariate analysis, left atrial size and class II symptoms at study entry were independent predictors for progression of heart failure symptoms to classes III/IV. Mortality was mainly due to progression of heart failure, with around 5% of deaths due to sudden cardiac deaths. But these 5% had refused intracardiac defibrillator (ICD) implantation.

Symptomatic permanent or paroxysmal atrial fibrillation (AF) occurred in 19% of non-obstructive patients, including 11% with previous history of AF, and 8% developed new-onset AF during follow-up, exclusive of arrhythmia occurring in the first 30 days following myectomy.

Left atrial size in these patients exceeded that in the patients without AF (44 ± 7.4 mm vs. 39 ± 6.6 mm; p < 0.001). Those with permanent AF underwent ablation by pulmonary vein isolation. Out of these patients, 2% had a thrombo-embolic stroke, though they had refused anticoagulation treatment.

On cardiac magnetic resonance (CMR) study, one or more areas of LGE, not confined to a coronary arterial vascular territory, were present in 68 patients (52%), occupying 7.1 ± 9.8% of LV myocardial volume, particularly marked (≥ 15%) in 8 patients (6%). The extent of LGE at study entry in non-obstructive patients who developed classes III/IV heart failure (and the percentage of patients with extensive LGE ≥ 15%) exceeded that in patients who remained in classes I/II over the follow-up period (15% vs. 6%; p = 0.01 and 38% vs. 3%; p < 0.001, respectively).

THE NATURAL HISTORY OF NON-OBSTRUCTIVE HCM AND OBSTRUCTIVE HCM

Compared with patients with a resting or provocable obstruction, non-obstructive patients had a lower EF and a smaller left atrial dimension, but a larger LV cavity size, and were more likely to show LGE on contrast-enhanced CMR. The progression of heart failure symptoms from classes I/II to III/IV was significantly less common in patients with non-obstructive HCM (i.e., 10%; 1.6%/year), compared with patients with a resting (38%; 7.4%/year; p < 0.001) or provocable obstruction (20%; 3.2%/year; p = 0.002). Atrial Fibrillation, before or after the initial visit, occurred in 19% of patients with non-obstructive HCM, less than in those with a resting obstruction (33%; p = 0.007), but not different from patients with a provocable obstruction (23%; p = 0.36). The occurrence of thrombo-embolic stroke was similar between patients with non-obstructive (2%) and obstructive (resting 2%; provocable 1%; p = 0.73) HCM. The HCM-related mortality rate in non-obstructive patients was low at 0.5%/year, with five and ten-year survival rates free of HCM death at 99% and 97% (95% CI: 97% to 99% and 95% to 98%, respectively), not different from patients with a resting (0.4%/year) or provocable obstruction (0.2%/year) (p = 0.48).

Sudden death, resuscitated out-of-hospital cardiac arrest, and appropriate ICD interventions for ventricular tachycardia/ventricular fibrillation (VF) occurred in 5.6% (0.9%/year) of non-obstructive patients, which is also similar to patients with a resting obstruction (0.6%/year) or provocable obstruction (0.8%/year; p = 0.51). Total mortality did not differ significantly among patients with non-obstructive HCM (0.9%/year) compared with those with a resting (1.0%/year) or provocable obstruction (0.5%/year; p = 0.39).

Patients with an outflow obstruction had a five-fold greater risk of developing debilitating symptoms and, notably, more than 90% of obstructive patients achieved a marked improvement in heart failure symptoms following relief of the subaortic gradient and normalization of LV pressures with myectomy (or, alternatively, alcohol septal ablation).

This observation underscores the principle that heart failure due to outflow obstruction is a treatable (and reversible) complication of HCM for which there is also a survival benefit.

However, this study identified a small subset of non-obstructive HCM patients (4%) who developed progressive and unrelenting heart failure symptoms that were refractory to pharmacological treatment and who required (or were considered for) heart transplantation as the only available therapeutic option with the potential to restore an acceptable quality of life. These transplant candidates constituted two distinct subgroups, including those with impaired systolic function and various degrees of adverse LV remodeling (i.e., regression of hypertrophy and ventricular chamber enlargement due to diffuse LV scarring), as well as patients with preserved EF, demonstrating little or no remodeling [20–22]. These latter patients represent a novel subgroup with non-obstructive disease, given that a seemingly large proportion of HCM transplant candidates in this cohort (i.e., 50%) did not meet the arbitrary EF cutoff for systolic dysfunction.

Those patients who develop advanced progressive heart failure, despite preserved systolic function, expand the spectrum of end-stage heart failure beyond LV systolic dysfunction. The choice to pursue transplantation in HCM patients with class III symptoms and preserved systolic function is challenging and requires taking into account individual clinical profiles (including results of metabolic exercise testing and invasive hemodynamic data), but ultimately the greatest weight is given to the clinical history and symptom profile. The basis of the decision to offer heart transplantation to such patients is the recognition that this is the only therapeutic option capable of restoring an acceptable quality of life and longevity to this subgroup of patients [21, 22].

CONCLUSIONS

Non-obstructive HCM patients comprise about one-third of the broad HCM hemodynamic spectrum. They appear to be at a relatively lower risk of developing most HCM-related complications, including progressive drug-refractory heart failure, sudden death, or embolic stroke, and have an HCM-related mortality rate of 0.5%/year (albeit with a small risk of heart transplantation).

Obstructive HCM has a worse prognosis in terms of progression to advanced heart failure and the need for prophylactic ICD. However, heart failure due to outflow obstruction is an eminently treatable (and reversible) complication of HCM. Myectomy or alcohol septal ablation also has a definite survival benefit.

REFERENCES

1. Maron BJ, Tajik AJ, Ruttenberg HD, Graham TP, Atwood GF, Victoria BE, Lie JT, Roberts WC. Hypertrophic cardiomyopathy in infants: clinical features and natural history. *Circulation* 1982; 65:7–17.
2. Fay WP, Taliercio CP, Ilstrup DM, Tajik AJ, Gersh BJ. Natural history of hypertrophic cardiomyopathy in the elderly. *J Am Coll Cardiol* 1990; 16:821–826.

3. Maron BJ, Spirito P, Wesley Y, Arce J. Development or progression of left ventricular hypertrophy in children with hypertrophic cardiomyopathy: identification by two-dimensional echocardiography. *N Engl J Med* 1986; 315:610–614.

4. Panza JA, Maris TJ, Maron BJ. Development and determinants of dynamic obstruction to left ventricular outflow in young patients with hypertrophic cardiomyopathy. *J Am Coll Cardiol* 1989;13:820–823.

5. Spirito P, Maron BJ. Absence of progression of left ventricular hypertrophy in adult patients with hypertrophic cardiomyopathy. *Am J Cardiol* 1987;9: 1013–1017.

6. Spirito P, Maron BJ, Bonow RO, Epstein SE. Occurrence and significance of progressive left ventricular wall thinning and relative cavity dilatation in patients with hypertrophic cardiomyopathy. *Am J Cardiol* 1987;60: 123–129.

7. Pastemac A, Noble J, Steulens Y, Elie R, Henschke C, Bourassa MG. Pathophysiology of chest pain in patients with cardiomyopathies and normal coronary arteries. *Circulation* 1982;65:778–789.

8. Cannon RO, Rosing DR, Maron BJ, Leon MB, Bonow RO, Watson RM, Epstein SE. Myocardial ischemia in patients with hypertrophic cardiomyopathy: contribution of inadequate vasodilator reserve and elevated left ventricular filling pressures. *Circulation* 1985;71:234–243.

9. O'Gara PT, Bonow RO, Maron BJ, et al. Myocardial perfusion abnormalities in patients with hypertrophic cardiomyopathy: assessment with thallium-201 emission computed tomography. *Circulation* 1987;76: 1214–1223.

10. Maron BJ, Wolfson JK, Epstein SE, Roberts WC. Intramural ("small vessel") coronary artery disease in hypertrophic cardiomyopathy. *J Am Coil Cardiol* 1986; 8:545–557.

11. McKenna WJ, Deanfield J, Faruqui A, England D, Oakley CM, Goodwin JF. Prognosis in hypertrophic cardiomyopathy: role of age, and clinical, electrocardiographic and hemodynamic features. *Am J Cardiol* 1981;47: 532–538.

12. Wingle ED, Sasson Z, Henderson MA, et al. Hypertrophic cardiomyopathy: the importance of the site and the extent of hypertrophy: a review. *Prog Cardiovasc Dis* 1985;28: 1–83.

13. Maron BJ, Bonow RO, Cannon RO III, Leon MB, Epstein SE. Hypertrophic cardiomyopathy: interrelations of clinical manifestations, pathophysiology, and therapy. *N Engl J Med* 1987;316:780–789, 844–852.

14. Maron MS, Maron BJ, Harrigan C, et al. Hypertrophic cardiomyopathy phenotype revisited after 50 years with cardiovascular magnetic resonance. *J Am Coll Cardiol* 2009;54:220–228.

15. Maron BJ, Ommen SR, Semsarian C, Spirito P, Olivotto I, Maron MS. Hypertrophic cardiomyopathy: present and future, with translation into contemporary cardiovascular medicine. *J Am Coll Cardiol* 2014;64:83–99.

16. Gersh BJ, Maron BJ, Bonow RO, et al. 2011 ACCF/AHA guideline for the diagnosis and treatment of hypertrophic cardiomyopathy: a report of the American College of Cardiology Foundation/American Heart Association Task Force on Practice Guidelines. *J Am Coll Cardiol* 2011;58:e212–e260.

17. Maron BJ, McKenna WJ, Danielson GK, et al. American College of Cardiology/European Society of Cardiology clinical expert consensus document on hypertrophic cardiomyopathy: a report of the American College of Cardiology Foundation Task Force on Clinical Expert Consensus Documents and the European Society of Cardiology Committee for Practice Guidelines. *J Am Coll Cardiol* 2003;42:1687–1713.

18. Liu Q, Li D, Berger AE, Johns RA, Gao L. Survival and prognostic factors in hypertrophic cardiomyopathy: a meta-analysis. *Sci Rep* 2017;7: 11957. doi: 10.1038/s41598-017-12289.

19. Maron MS, Rowin EJ, Olivotto I, Casey SA, Arretini A, Tomberli B, Garberich RF, Link MS, Chan RHM, Lesser JR, Maron BJ. Contemporary natural history and management of nonobstructive hypertrophic cardiomyopathy. *J Am Coll Cardiol* 2016;67:1399–1409.

20. Fernández A, Vigliano CA, Casabé JH, et al. Comparison of prevalence, clinical course, and pathological findings of left ventricular systolic impairment versus normal systolic function in patients with hypertrophic cardiomyopathy. *Am J Cardiol* 2011;108:548–555.
21. Rowin EJ, Maron BJ, Kiernan MS, et al. Advanced heart failure with preserved systolic function in nonobstructive hypertrophic cardiomyopathy: under-recognized subset of candidates for heart transplant. *Circ Heart Fail* 2014;7: 967–975.
22. Pasqualucci D, Fornaro A, Castelli G, et al. Clinical spectrum, therapeutic options, and outcome of advanced heart failure in hypertrophic cardiomyopathy. *Circ Heart Fail* 2015;8:1014–1021.

Chapter 4

ECHOCARDIOGRAPHIC FEATURES OF HYPERTROPHIC CARDIOMYOPATHY

Satish C. Govind

CONTENTS

Table 4.1   Echocardiography in HCM

Echocardiography	Utility
Trans-thoracic	• Initial diagnostic test • Monitoring /follow-up purposes • Screening test of family members
Tissue Doppler imaging	• Sub clinical systolic regional abnormalities • Left ventricular diastolic function assessment
Speckle tracking echocardiography	• Left ventricular systolic function assessment by global longitudinal strain • Identification of regional segments affected by fibrosis
3D echocardiography	• Localization of anatomic abnormalities • Volume estimation of left ventricle and left atrium
Contrast echocardiography	• Confirmation of apical aneurysm and apical hypertrophic cardiomyopathy • Septal ablation
Exercise echocardiography	• Evaluation of symptomatic patients having no significant obstruction at rest
Transesophageal echocardiography	• Peri-operative role during myectomy • Mitral valve evaluation

INTRODUCTION

Hypertrophic cardiomyopathy (HCM), an inherited complex myocardial disease, can be quite diverse in its presentation. It is characterized by myocardial hypertrophy, patchy interstitial fibrosis, myocardial fiber disarray, ventricular dysfunction, and other structural and hemodynamic abnormalities [1]. Historically, ventricular hypertrophy and other abnormal findings of HCM have been imaged using conventional echocardiography comprising M-mode, 2D, and Doppler applications. These applications are complementary to each other, with 2D echocardiography (2DE) providing anatomic information, while the Doppler study contributes to the hemodynamic data. This non-invasive test, a first-line imaging modality, is used extensively not just in the diagnosis of HCM but also as a screening test for families of affected individuals, in guiding interventional procedures, and in the monitoring and follow-up of patients. Advances, such as tissue Doppler imaging (TDI), contrast echocardiography, speckle tracking echocardiography (STE), and 3D echocardiography (3DE), have boosted echocardiographic imaging's capabilities and made it an invaluable imaging tool in diagnostic and management protocols [2]. Transesophageal echocardiography (TEE) and exercise echocardiography are special procedures that are less used but have important roles to play in select scenarios.

Guidelines on HCM published by various societies [3–6] around the world emphasize the importance of trans-thoracic echocardiography and recommend it as a frontline test. It is a class I investigation for an initial test of patients suspected of having HCM. Subsequent testing forms a part of follow-up studies, as per protocol, or when there is a change in clinical status, or when a new cardiovascular event has occurred. Echocardiography in HCM has to be a methodical and comprehensive study, utilizing all available methods, both conventional and advanced applications (Table 4.1).

Imaging objectives should focus on [2, 7]:

● Description of hypertrophy patterns in the left ventricle (LV) and right ventricle (RV);
● Septal morphology;
● Mitral valve (MV) abnormalities;
● Measuring ventricular gradients in LV and RV for the presence of significant obstruction;

- Evaluation of mitral regurgitation (MR);
- LV function assessment;
- Detection of LV apical abnormalities;
- Identifying associated lesions.

Decisions about the need for additional imaging are made after initial trans-thoracic echocardiography has been done.

PATTERNS OF VENTRICULAR HYPERTROPHY

The characteristic feature of HCM is a non-dilated LV and an unexplained left ventricular hypertrophy (LVH), presenting in the absence of another disease that may cause hypertrophy. Left ventricular wall thickness is increased, ranging from mild to severe hypertrophy. Morphologic variabilities of HCM, as seen in 2DE, has led to many classifications, the most accepted being the Maron classification [8] (Table 4.2).

Left ventricular hypertrophy is highly variable in HCM (Figures 4.1 and 4.2), ranging from the classical asymmetrical type to rarer variants involving isolated walls but sparing the interventricular septum (IVS). Hypertrophic cardiomyopathy is marked by areas of hypertrophy with intervening normal LV thickness (almost one-half of patients show many segments of normal LV thickness). Fifteen percent of individuals show the involvement of one to two segments (LV mass can be normal in this subset), while patterns of symmetric hypertrophy are seen less often. The finding is usually that of asymmetric LVH, with the anteroseptum commonly affected and having the maximal thickness, especially at the junction where the anteroseptum transitions into the anterior wall (overestimation of thickness occurs when the RV side of the septal thickness is inadvertently included). The more proximal the hypertrophy, the higher the association of outflow obstruction.

M-MODE ECHOCARDIOGRAPHY

This modality is the oldest in terms of its application, but is still relevant and of great utility in present-day echo assessment of HCM [9]. The superior temporal resolution makes it perfect for observing the timing of events during the cardiac cycle. Measurements are often made from a good parasternal long-axis view using appropriate sweep speeds (50–100 mm/s). It is frequently used in identifying the presence and severity of systolic anterior motion (SAM) of the mitral valve (MV), premature closure of the aortic valve (mid-systolic notching), and also for measuring IVS and LV posterior wall thickness. A major limitation of M-mode echocardiography is that non-perpendicular measurements lead to erroneous values and misinterpretations.

TWO-DIMENSIONAL ECHOCARDIOGRAPHY

The diagnosis of HCM is established most often by two-dimensional echocardiography (2DE) and is the cornerstone in imaging of the various associated structural abnormalities. It provides for real-time imaging of the structures, observing myocardial texture, and for making measurements. Imaging includes locating the distribution of hypertrophy, whether it is diffuse or segmental, whether there is asymmetric or symmetric thickening, and measuring the maximal

Table 4.2   Maron classification of patterns of LVH based on 2DE

Type	Morphologic variability
I	LVH (usually mild) involving anterior part of interventricular septum
II	LVH involving anterior and posterior part of interventricular septum
III	LVH involving anterior and posterior part of interventricular septum plus anterolateral free wall
IV	Unusual patterns of LVH (anterior part of interventricular septum is spared)

(A)

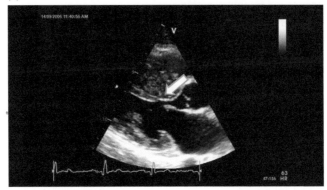

(B)

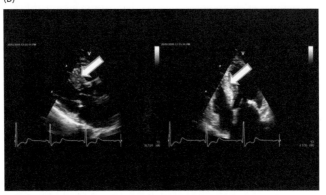

(C)

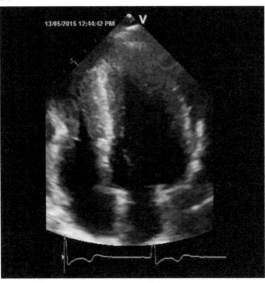

Figure 4.1 Varying patterns of HCM. (*A*) Anteroseptum is hypertrophied (white arrow), with normal thickness of the LV posterior wall. (*B*) Anteroseptum and inferoseptum are both hypertrophied (white arrows), with normal thickness of LV posterior and lateral wall. (*C*) Inferoseptum and lateral wall are both hypertrophied.

(A)

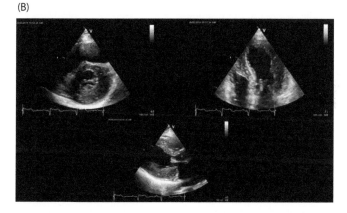

(B)

(C)

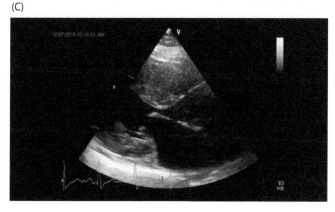

Figure 4.2 Unusual variations of HCM. (*A*) Symmetrical hypertrophy of the LV. (*B*) Posterior, lateral, and anterior wall grossly hypertrophied with only mild hypertrophy of the septum. (*C*) Both basal anteroseptum and LV posterior wall are significantly hypertrophied.

thickness using multiple views and multiple levels. HCM assessment by echocardiography requires meticulous imaging using multiple imaging planes (parasternal, apical, and also off-axis views) with optimal beam alignment to avoid oblique planes for identifying LVH, especially subtle segmental hypertrophy. Besides, a proper understanding of the principles of echo and knobology is needed for LVH identification and accurate measurements of wall thickness.

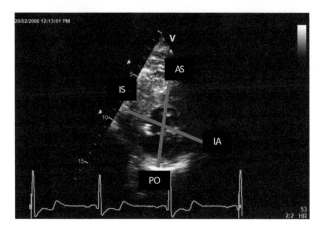

Figure 4.3 Parasternal short-axis view of the LV is shown where measurements of LV wall thickness can be made. IS, inferoseptum; AS, anteroseptum; PO, posterior; LA, lateral.

A simple but effective way of looking at LVH distribution and thickness measurement is by way of 2DE images in the parasternal short-axis view (Figure 4.3), where LV cross-sectional images can be analyzed at multiple levels [10].

HYPERTROPHIED LEFT VENTRICLE

Classically, an LV wall thickness at end-diastole of more than 15 mm (average of 20 mm) and an IVS to posterior wall-thickness ratio of more than 1.3 with no other cause for hypertrophy is considered to be HCM [9, 11]. Measurements of 13–15 mm are the gray zone areas and need to be combined with genetic testing after excluding the athlete's heart or hypertensive heart disease. Severe wall thickness of more than 30 mm should specifically be looked for, since it is associated with arrhythmias and sudden cardiac death (the basal septum is the segment frequently involved, measured, and also the easiest to image). Left ventricular wall thickness of 12–15 mm in relatives of an affected individual is indicative of HCM [12].

Occasionally, the anterior and lateral wall of the LV and the LV apex is not optimally imaged due to technical challenges or poor imaging windows. In such situations, contrast echocardiography can be an alternative for better visualization of these structures [13]. In suspected individuals with minimal LVH, elongated mitral leaflets, papillary muscle (PPM) thickening, and accessory muscle bundles are clues to the presence of HCM. Infrequently HCM may coexist with other cardiac diseases such as coronary artery disease, aortic valve disease (Figure 4.4), and congenital heart disease. Comprehensive echocardiography requires that such conditions are identified along with HCM findings, despite HCM masking some classic findings of these diseases.

NON-HYPERTROPHIED LEFT VENTRICLE

It should be noted that not all patients with HCM demonstrate LVH, especially children below the age of 13 [11]. The appearance and progressive increase of LVH are seen as children transition from adolescence into adulthood. Mutations of the gene, myosin-binding protein C, has been linked to this delayed appearance of LVH in adults [14, 15]. This type of genotype positive, with no LVH, can also present with prominent invaginations of the basal IVS and the anterolateral wall (myocardial crypts). Widespread genetic testing has recently identified an expanding subset (adults and children) of HCM where mutation of the gene results in the absence of LVH early on in the disease has led to situations where many issues are yet to be resolved. Hence, if LVH is absent on echo at index presentation, even in adults, it is important to follow up and periodically screen these individuals who are genotype positive, as well as the family members, to detect late-onset HCM. The limitation of 2DE is its

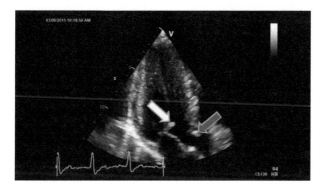

Figure 4.4 Hypertrophic cardiomyopathy with systolic anterior motion of the mitral leaflet with narrowed LV outflow tract (white arrow). There is an associated unusual involvement of the aortic valve with thickened leaflets and mildly restricted mobility (red arrow).

inability to detect subtle regional hypertrophy in suboptimal imaging windows and at-risk individuals who have genetic abnormality but do not clinically and echocardiographically manifest.

APICAL HCM

Apical HCM (Figure 4.5) is more sporadic (one can term it as infrequent, rather than rare) and has a wide spectrum of presentation. It is generally defined as an apical wall thickness of more than 13–15 mm or an apical to posterior wall-thickness ratio of more than 1.5, with associated loss of normal apical contour or tapering [16], giving a spade-like appearance of the LV cavity.

Three phenotypic types are broadly described [16, 17]:

- Pure: isolated apical hypertrophy;
- Mixed: apical and IVS hypertrophy;
- Relative: minimal apical thickening (earliest manifestation) which progresses to overt hypertrophy with time.

Other features of apical HCM are dilated left atrium (LA), apical aneurysm, cavity obliteration at the apex, and mid-cavity obstruction. Apical cavity obliteration is more likely with the pure type. Interestingly, the ratio measured of the end-systolic length of the obliterated apex segment to that of the end-systolic length of the rest of the LV cavity, a ratio of more than 0.5, suggests increased cardiac adverse events. Mid-cavity obstruction is more likely with mixed types of apical HCM, where the hypertrophied IVS makes contact with a

(A)   (B)

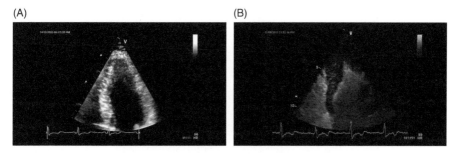

Figure 4.5 Apical HCM. (A) Non-contrast filled LV. (B) Contrast opacified LV showing markedly improved image quality, with excellent delineation of the apical hypertrophy (note the "spade-shaped" LV cavity).

vigorously contracting normal-thickness lateral wall in the presence of hypertrophied PPM. Mistaking focal thickening of the LV apex or apically displaced PPM or the presence of accessory muscle bundles can lead to an erroneous diagnosis of apical HCM on 2DE when viewed from a tangential plane. There is no LV outflow tract obstruction (LVOTO) or related MR seen in apical HCM.

SEPTAL HYPERTROPHY

Interventricular septum is frequently affected in HCM with varying morphology. The shape of the IVS has been shown to have an impact on clinical outcomes. The reverse septum type has been associated with younger age groups, having greater LV mass, more advanced disease, more adverse remodeling, and a higher burden of fibrosis. This group has been identified as high risk with a propensity for sudden cardiac death.

The following types of septal morphology have been described based on trans-thoracic echocardiography [2]:

- Reverse curvature or catenoid septum: mid-IVS is convex towards the LV cavity. Maximal thickness is seen at mid-IVS (apical four-chamber view).
- Sigmoid septum: IVS is concave to the LV cavity due to the pronounced basal septal hypertrophy. Maximal thickness is seen at basal IVS (parasternal long-axis and apical four-chamber views).
- Neutral septum: IVS is straight since it is uniformly thickened. The ratio of maximal IVS thickness to each segment is > 0.8 (apical four-chamber view).
- Apical septum: Maximal IVS thickness is seen in the apical segment (apical four-chamber view).

RIGHT VENTRICULAR HYPERTROPHY

Right ventricular hypertrophy (more than 8 mm) is known to be associated with LV HCM in about one-third of patients [18]. This involvement has been described as the presence of two or more hypertrophied segments, but it often presents diffuse involvement affecting three segments. Right ventricular outflow tract (RVOT) obstruction is also seen (Figure 4.6), either in association with LVOTO or in isolation [19]. Right ventricular outflow tract RVOT hypertrophy is frequently involved with HCM of the LV, seen in almost half of the patients. Low spatial resolution, the complex geometry of the RV, and suboptimal echocardiography

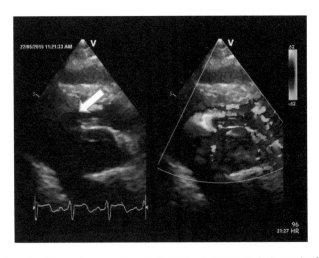

Figure 4.6 Hypertrophic cardiomyopathy with RVOT involvement. Turbulent color flow is seen at RVOT, at the site of the obstruction.

windows prevent abnormalities being detected clearly, especially mild changes. Apart from its unusual geometry, its location, presence of epicardial fat adjacent to the free wall, and prominent trabeculations, the RV poses challenges during echocardiography, many a time providing inconclusive information. Difficult echo windows further hinder a good examination of the RV. There is limited information on RV HCM in published data.

VENTRICULAR HYPERTROPHY DUE TO OTHER CAUSES

Some conditions which present as LVH or biventricular hypertrophy lead to diagnostic dilemmas as to whether it is HCM or some other hypertrophic condition, or uncommonly there may be an overlap of both. Some of these conditions commonly encountered in routine practice are an athlete's heart, hypertensive disease, Fabry's disease, and other infiltrative disorders. The athlete's heart [2, 20] has only a mild increase in LV size (more than 55 mm), while HCM typically has a non-dilated LV (size less than 45 mm). Left ventricular wall or IVS thickness in HCM is more than 15 mm, reaching up to 30 mm, while in athlete's heart it is usually less than 15 mm with a lack of LVH regression after cessation of exercise. The presence of pericardial effusion and a low voltage electrocardiogram are in favor of Fabry's disease. An IVS to LV posterior wall-thickness ratio of more than 1.5:1, the presence of asymmetrical LV wall thickening with normal thickness in some LV segments, an LV wall thickness of more than 18 mm, and the presence of MV abnormalities provide a clue as to the presence of HCM. Diagnostic challenges unresolved by echocardiography may require further testing with other imaging modalities to establish the cause of LVH.

THE MITRAL VALVE

Hypertrophic cardiomyopathy is associated with an abnormal MV in the majority of patients, where it can involve one or more components of the MV complex (leaflets, chordae, and papillary muscles) [21]. Over the last few decades, there has been an increased focus on MV structural abnormalities, its role in LVOTO, management planning when procedural interventions are strategized, and while evaluating clinical outcomes. In this era of MV repair, where the objective is to salvage the native valve to whatever extent possible, it is vital that the echocardiographer has sufficient knowledge of MV anatomy and the various abnormalities associated with HCM. Special attention is required in individuals with a lesser degree of IVS hypertrophy or LVH, but with LVOTO present, where MV abnormalities play an important mechanistic role.

The structural abnormality first noticed in the early years of scientific work on LVOTO was an anteriorly displaced MV (specifically the papillary muscles) impeding the flow being ejected out of the LV. Papillary muscle abnormalities are seen as either hypertrophied structures or the presence of an anomalous PPM or direct attachment of the PPM to the mitral leaflets [21]. However, the main components of MV involved are the leaflets, where the common abnormality is an elongated anterior mitral leaflet (AML), and occasionally an elongated posterior mitral leaflet (PML). Chordal abnormalities present as lax chordae or a short chordae or sometimes even its absence. Mitral leaflet or annular calcification, when present, is usually associated with significant SAM.

The following MV changes predispose to LVOTO:

- Papillary muscle positioned anteriorly towards IVS – correspondingly, the coaptation plane moves anteriorly;
- Abnormal papillary muscle thickening;
- Anomalous papillary muscle having a direct attachment to the mid-AML;
- Elongated mitral leaflets;
- Anomalous chordal attachment to the leaflets;
- Chordal fibrosis.

LEAFLETS

The AML is elongated in most HCM patients (it is less than 30 mm in healthy subjects) and is even more pronounced in patients with LVOTO with an average length of 34–35 mm (measurement includes the aorto-mitral area), with the coapted leaflets having an average extension of 24 mm below the level of the mitral annulus during systole [21]. Frequently the tip of the AML beyond the coaptation point curves into the left ventricular outflow tract (LVOT) and this small length of the leaflet is influenced by the bloodstream rather than the chamber pressures and leans towards or touches the IVS causing LVOTO. Corrective surgical procedures of the mitral leaflets are based on these mechanics and the abnormal measurements obtained during imaging. Isolated PML elongation (the length is less than 15–17 mm in healthy subjects) is infrequently seen, but when present can contribute to LVOTO. The cause of the elongation of leaflets has been attributed to a primary phenotypic manifestation and not due to any secondary stretch factors of an anteriorly displaced MV. It is important to note that elongation of leaflets is not due to any myxomatous changes, but are elongated cell lines originating from the coelomic mesothelium (though concomitant myxomatous disease has also been reported in some patients, which may add to the complexity of the disease).

PAPILLARY MUSCLES

Papillary muscle abnormalities are seen frequently, appearing as hypertrophy (this occurs in > 50% of HCM individuals) and as a structure displaced from its usual anatomical location. The reported standard end-diastolic width or thickness in the parasternal short-axis view of PPM is less than 11 mm, while the standard length is about 30 mm [22]. Mid-cavity obstruction of the LV occurs by contact of the thickened anterior PPM with the IVS. Thickened PPM is also associated with an abnormal fusion anteriorly to the ventricular wall (Figures 4.7 and 4.8) and as a projection into the LV cavity, with both PPM facing each other, thus reducing the distance between the PPM's leading to outflow obstruction. Another characteristic feature seen is a displaced PPM, usually involving the anterior PPM. One should be careful not to mistake an apically displaced PPM as apical HCM. Anomalous and bifid PPM (seen from a parasternal short-axis view as an anteriorly located muscle mass) are abnormalities frequently seen and which are also a frequent cause of LVOTO, as they increase in thickness over time. Direct insertion of the anterior PPM into the mid-AML can be imaged fairly well using parasternal long-axis and apical views (Figure 4.9) or off-axis views. However, echocardiographic imaging becomes a challenge when the direct insertion is located close to the anterolateral commissure.

(A)   (B)

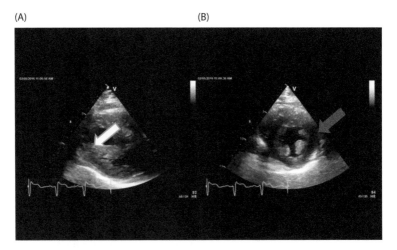

Figure 4.7 (A) Parasternal long-axis view of hypertrophied papillary muscle (white arrow). (B) Parasternal short-axis view of thickened papillary muscles with an accessory anterolateral papillary muscle (red arrow).

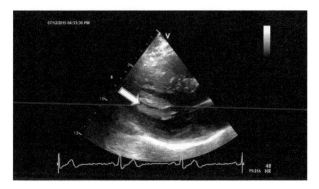

Figure 4.8 Parasternal long-axis view of hypertrophied papillary muscles (white arrow) and an accessory muscle band (red arrow).

(A)   (B)

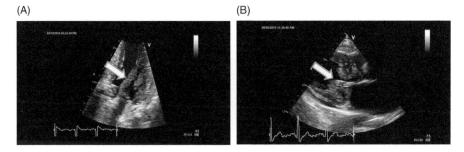

Figure 4.9 Direct insertion of papillary muscle into anterior mitral leaflet. (*A*) Apical four-chamber view. (*B*) Parasternal long-axis view.

Three-dimensional echocardiography (3DE) can be a useful tool in such situations with a higher detection rate. Other interesting findings noticed in HCM are that of a bifid PPM with increased mobility and accessory muscle bundles coursing from the apex to the basal IVS or anterior basal wall, again a cause of LVOTO.

CHORDAE
Chordal abnormalities are also a cause of LVOTO, in the form of fibrotic or retracted chordae [21, 22]. They cause tenting of the MV and displace it anteriorly towards the LVOT. Spontaneous rupture of chordae has also been reported in some individuals with HCM, leading to significant MR.

LEFT VENTRICULAR OBSTRUCTION

Hypertrophic cardiomyopathy can be termed as either non-obstructive or obstructive and defined as a resting peak gradient of more than 30 mm Hg. In about 30% of HCM patients, obstruction is seen at rest, while in 40%, it is detected after provocative maneuvers, while the remaining one-third of patients are non-obstructive [11, 23]. Peak gradients of more than 50 mm Hg represent a category where interventions can be considered. Apart from LVOTO, the obstruction can present at different levels within the LV cavity.

When the resting Doppler peak gradients are not indicative of obstruction, provocative maneuvers are applied to elicit what are called "provocable gradients" to confirm the presence or absence of obstruction [11, 23]. Commonly, the Valsalva maneuver, or making the individual stand up, are employed when assessing gradients (successful in about 50% of patients).

Alternatively, pharmacological interventions such as amyl nitrite with two to three inhalations over two minutes (moderately reliable) or dobutamine or isoproterenol (unreliable due to high false positives) have been described as methods to induce gradients. They are generally used when physiological maneuvers are not possible or when they were unsuccessful. The appearance of a ventricular premature beat (VPB) is also utilized during echocardiography, wherein a post-VPB Doppler gradient can be reflective of either the absence or presence of an underlying obstruction. Ideally, both resting and provocable gradients should always be reported on echocardiography.

DOPPLER EVALUATION

Doppler imaging plays an invaluable role in the assessment of HCM [23, 24]. A comprehensive Doppler study includes color-flow evaluation, pulsed-wave (PWD), and continuous-wave Doppler imaging (CWD).

COLOR-FLOW IMAGING

This contributes to initial information about a possible presence of obstruction (Figures 4.10 and 4.11), where a flow acceleration and turbulence, when seen, indicates obstruction either at the LVOT or at any level within the ventricular cavity (later quantified by PWD or CWD). It is

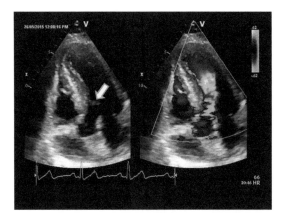

Figure 4.10 Hypertrophic cardiomyopathy with only LVOT involvement. Turbulent color flow seen at LVOT, where the obstruction is present. Systolic anterior motion of the mitral valve is seen (white arrow). Note that no obstruction is present at the mid-cavity and apex.

(A)   (B)

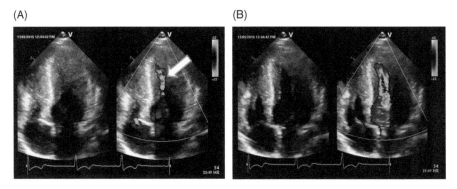

Figure 4.11 HCM with only mid-ventricular and apical involvement of two different patients. (*A*) Turbulent color flow (white arrow) with a slit-like LV cavity seen from mid-level to apex. (*B*) Note that no obstruction is seen at the basal septum in both patients.

also useful in detecting MR, its severity, and observing the direction of the regurgitant jet so as to understand its mechanism.

PULSED-WAVE DOPPLER IMAGING

Pulsed-wave Doppler imaging (PWD) allows for sampling the flow at a particular point in the LV to localize a high velocity obstructed flow [9]. When the obstruction is suspected at multiple levels, it can help to localize the level of obstruction. The LV cavity is systematically investigated by moving the PWD sampling, starting from the aortic valve, then moving it across to the LVOT and further into the mid-cavity and going all the way to the apex when required. A well-known finding of PWD is the so-called "lobster claw" appearance of the waveform in severe LVOTO (peak gradiant [PG] > 60 mm Hg), where rapid afterload changes lead to a series of events in systole. A quickly decelerating flow stream with reduced velocity is seen in early systole, followed by the sudden deceleration of the flow in mid-systole due to the obstruction, with late systole showing reappearance of the flow as the obstruction is released.

One has to be aware that PWD is open to measurement errors: It cannot assess velocities exceeding the Nyquist limit, and when the obstruction is at multiple levels in the line of Doppler interrogation, one may not be successful in localizing the obstruction on some occasions due to technical reasons. PWD usage, apart from its utility in assessing obstruction, is also helpful in the evaluation of diastolic function and, to a limited extent, as a supporting tool while grading the severity of MR.

CONTINUOUS-WAVE DOPPLER IMAGING

Continuous-wave Doppler imaging (CWD), unlike PWD, is capable of measuring high gradients and is the method of choice when evaluating severe obstruction since the principle of the Nyquist limit does not apply when using it [25]. The characteristic feature of a dynamic obstruction in HCM is a Doppler waveform that resembles a dagger (the concavity seen on one side of the Doppler waveform) which happens because of poor early systolic flow, followed by the appearance of a mid-systolic acceleration, and culminating with a late systolic peaking. This has to be differentiated from an MR or an aortic stenosis (AS) jet. An MR jet is holosystolic and symmetrical, with a peak velocity of usually more than 6 m/s, having a longer duration (it involves both iso-volumic phases), and having a parabolic curving at its peak. A fixed obstruction like AS has an early to mid-systolic peaking of the Doppler waveform depending on its severity.

One must be cautious when interpreting the obtained gradient value since severity can be underestimated if the line of Doppler interrogation is not parallel to the flow of blood; it can also be overestimated if the Doppler cursor overlaps an MR jet which leads to high gradients being erroneously interpreted as severe obstruction. Often, the LVOTO Doppler waveform can be hidden or can be faintly visible within an MR jet. Thus, to avoid such pitfalls, Doppler investigation has to be done from multiple views and planes, in line with the flow and with optimal gain settings to obtain reliable readings.

LEFT VENTRICULAR OUTFLOW TRACT OBSTRUCTION

Left ventricular outflow tract obstruction is seen more often than LV mid-cavity obstruction. It has been the hallmark of obstructive HCM since the early descriptions of the latter. It occurs in the presence of SAM (Figures 4.12 and 4.13) and a bulging basal IVS, which causes narrowing of the outflow tract, or contact of the MV with the IVS is made. A narrowed outflow tract characterizes the milder form, while a more severe degree is characterized by prolonged contact of a part of the MV with the IVS at mid- to late systole, causing flow obstruction and diminished stroke volume.

SYSTOLIC ANTERIOR MOTION OF THE MITRAL VALVE

The severity of SAM is generally graded as:

- Grade 1: when the MV has not made any contact with the IVS, but the measured distance from the IVS is more than 10 mm.
- Grade 2 (mild): when the MV has not made any contact with the IVS, but the measured distance from the IVS is less than 10 mm.

(A)   (B)

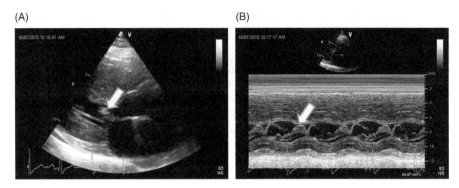

Figure 4.12 Parasternal long view showing hypertrophied septum and SAM of the MV with LVOTO (white arrows). (*A*) SAM seen on 2D. (*B*) SAM seen on M-mode.

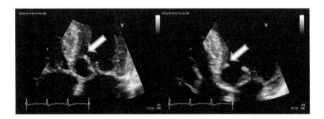

Figure 4.13 Repetitive contact of the anterior mitral leaflet with the septum over a long duration has resulted in a fibrotic area on the thickened basal septum (white arrow). This is the point of maximal flow obstruction.

- Grade 3 (moderate): when the MV makes contact with the IVS for a duration of less than 30% of systole.
- Grade 4 (severe): when the MV makes contact with the IVS for a duration of 30% of systole or more.

The AML is commonly involved in SAM [9] when contact is made with the IVS, but occasionally an unusually long PML [26] can also be attributed to SAM (5%). Two-dimensional echocardiography (parasternal long-axis or apical four-chamber views) is the preferred approach to observe SAM in real-time imaging and also to visualize the surrounding structures contributing to it. The effect of SAM leads to malcoaptation of the mitral leaflets, causing a characteristic MR jet, which is postero-laterally directed. Post-myectomy, once the LVOTO has reduced, such MRs decrease over time. If the MR jet is centrally or anteriorly directed, it invariably points to an intrinsic leaflet abnormality, like a prolapsed or a flail leaflet. In such instances, there may be a need for surgical intervention of MV to correct the MR in addition to septal myectomy.

The severity of flow obstruction is quantified by Doppler echocardiography. Left ventricular outflow tract obstruction has generated controversy, and been much debated and discussed over the years, with some areas still unclear when it comes to its clinical presentation and its mechanism. Two widely accepted mechanisms [11] for SAM have been the:

- Drag effect, where the anterior displacement of the MV increases the area of the AML to the forces of rapid blood flow along with IVS, which pulls or drags the MV towards the IVS. The LV blood flow postulation describes a thickened IVS with an LV ejection flow stream that exerts a force on the posterior side of the MV tips; pushing, it moves anteriorly, causing the early phase of SAM.
- Venturi effect, where a bulging basal septum causes pressure variation in LV outflow to draw or suck the mitral leaflets towards the LVOT.

Overall, the drag effect offers a better explanation of the mechanism of SAM. Another area of the debate has been about which of the two contributes most to SAM, with general acceptance being that both mechanisms are responsible for many patients.

Structurally, the predisposing factors for LVOTO are:

- Highly thickened antero-basal IVS;
- Narrowed LV outflow tract;
- A small LV cavity;
- Abnormal MV apparatus/SAM;
- A steep LV to aortic root angle (aorto-mitral angle is less than 120 degrees).

DYNAMIC GRADIENT

The majority of patients with HCM present with either obstruction at rest or show obstruction with provocation, while a lesser percentage has neither. Left ventricular outflow tract obstruction is very much a dynamic process [27], and the obstruction or the gradient is very much dependent on load: Decreased LV filling or increased LV contractility is characterized by increased gradient, while increased LV filling reduces the gradient. Left ventricular outflow tract gradients are extremely dynamic and variable to the extent that they can be influenced by volume, increased physical activity, the position of the patient, anesthetic and non-anesthetic medications, autonomic nervous system, heavy meals, and even alcohol. Higher gradients are seen after a heavy meal, while those on beta blockers may have lower gradients. This sort of gradient fluctuation, sometimes even seen in the setting of a single study, must be factored in when critical decisions are to be taken. In such situations, it is essential to perform provocative maneuvers, especially in symptomatic patients.

The Doppler waveform of LVOTO is characterized by flow acceleration in mid-systole (mid-third) with late systolic peaking (Figures 4.14 and 4.15) with loss of signal intensity as velocity increases. Flow acceleration seen during systole can be variable, where the flow sometimes can increase even at mid-systole, giving it a more symmetrical shape than the classic curvy late-peaking concave shape. A sigmoid septum causing LVOTO in the elderly is a separate entity and not to be confused with HCM since it is an age-related phenomenon.

MITRAL REGURGITATION

Mitral regurgitation (MR) in HCM is caused by inadequate coaptation of the mitral leaflets. The mismatched length and increased mobility of the leaflets (elongated AML and a PML unable to compensate in length and mobility) results in MR, which is postero-laterally directed (Figure 4.16), a classic finding in LVOTO. An anteriorly directed or central jet, on the other hand, can be due to PML prolapse or due to a mechanism caused by fibrosis, ruptured chordae, or calcification of the MV. It should be noted that a mid-cavity obstruction with no LVOTO or

(A)   (B)

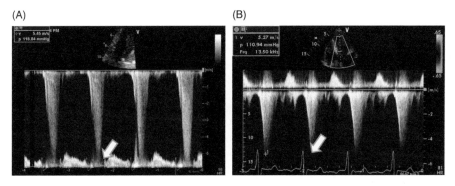

Figure 4.14 (A) Pulsed-wave Doppler showing aliasing of high velocity obstructive gradient. (B) Continuous-wave Doppler of a high velocity obstructive gradient with no aliasing.

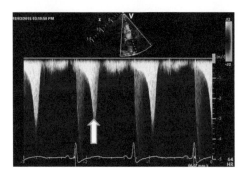

Figure 4.15 Dynamic obstruction with high gradient and characteristic concavity with late systolic peaking visible (note the dagger-shaped wave form).

(A)   (B)

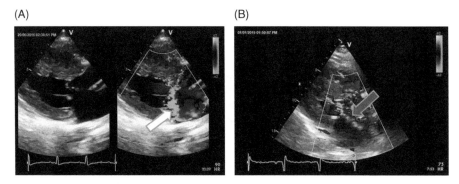

Figure 4.16 Parasternal long-axis views showing MR. (A) MR is posteriorly directed (white arrow) because of improper coaptation of leaflets characteristic of systolic anterior motion of the MV. (B) MR is anteriorly directed (red arrow), suggestive of intrinsic leaflet abnormality (a posterior mitral leaflet prolapse in this patient).

apical HCM causes a postero-laterally directed MR. Mitral regurgitation can vary from individual to individual, despite having the same severity of outflow obstruction. It may be directly proportional, that is, the more severe the obstruction, the more the MR severity increases proportionally. In others, while MR may not increase, it is attributed to structural changes in MV anatomy, especially the mitral leaflets, and more so, a proportionally lengthy PML attempting better coaptation with an elongated AML.

LEFT VENTRICULAR MID-CAVITY OBSTRUCTION
An HCM patient can have LVOTO alone or an LV mid-cavity obstruction alone or both. Mid-cavity obstruction of the LV is caused by a hypertrophied IVS (catenoid type), making contact with the anterolateral wall of the LV and the adjacent hypertrophied PPMs. Direct attachment of the anterior PPM into the AML is another cause, where it forms a rigid "bridge"-like structure pointed towards the IVS, predisposing it to mid-cavity obstruction. LV mid-cavity obstruction is seen in about 10% of HCM patients, and its presence predisposes it to a higher ventricular adverse remodeling with associated arrhythmias and heart failure [28]. Aneurysm of the LV apex is seen in about 25% of individuals with LV mid-cavity obstruction, and these aneurysms can harbor a thrombus with the potential for embolism. Unlike LVOTO, the Doppler waveform of a mid-cavity obstruction is generally seen in an

even later part of systole (i.e., after two-thirds of systole has happened) as it usually accelerates and peaks during this late phase.

LEFT VENTRICULAR APICAL ANEURYSM

Left ventricular apical aneurysm (transverse size may range from 10 mm to more than 60 mm) with normal epicardial coronary arteries is a complication that should always be looked for in LV mid-cavity obstruction or apical hypertrophy. Aneurysm happens due to prolonged exposure of the LV apex to increased LV wall stress and chronic myocardial ischemia. Typical features of this aneurysm (Figure 4.17) are a thin-walled and dyskinetic cavity that may have a thrombus (Figure 4.18) with the potential for stroke. The scarred wall of the cavity has been associated with adverse events like arrhythmias and sudden cardiac death [9]. Doppler sampling at the neck of the aneurysm usually demonstrates a typical biphasic pattern [29]. Early systole shows reduced velocity as the aneurysmal cavity makes an ineffectual contraction, with the rest of systole showing an absent signal (flow is retained in the aneurysm) due to mid-cavity obstruction followed by an early diastole flow as the aneurysm empties the retained residual flow. In suboptimal echocardiographic windows, use of a contrast agent has been shown to improve the detection of the apical aneurysm and also the presence or absence of a thrombus.

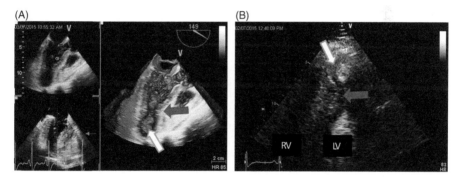

Figure 4.17 Left ventricular apical aneurysm (white arrows) with mid-cavity obstruction (red arrows) (both images of same patient). (A) Three-dimensional transesophageal echocardiogram of long axis of LV. (B) Trans-thoracic echocardiogram of apical four-chamber view showing contrast opacified LV.

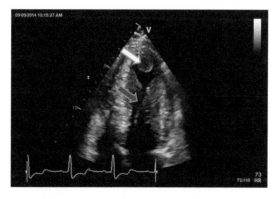

Figure 4.18 Apical four-chamber view showing mid-cavity obstruction of LV (red arrow) with aneurysm of apex and thrombus within it (white arrow).

SYSTOLIC FUNCTION

Systolic function quantification poses many challenges when using the widely used method of 2DE LV ejection fraction (LVEF) by way of a biplane-modified Simpson's approach [9]. A hyperdynamic LV or a small cavity with loss of chamber geometry and suboptimal imaging windows often leads to unreliable measurements. When LVEF is done correctly, a supranormal value of more than 70% is commonly encountered in patients with HCM, which does not necessarily reflect a supernormal healthy LV. A high LVEF does not truly reflect the underlying abnormal LV myocardial function since it is not sensitive enough to detect subtle changes occurring in the myocardium. Left ventricular ejection fraction is generally considered a poor measure of systolic function since radial contractility which is increased in the hypertrophied myocardium leads to a falsely high value of LVEF. However, worsening LVEF on serial monitoring may indicate a progression towards end-stage disease, with LVEF of less than 50% signaling adverse cardiac events. Progress to the end-stage phase presents mainly as a worsening systolic function (Figure 4.19) with LV dilatation and wall thinning seen in less than 50% of patients (LVH may continue to be seen in the end stage in some patients), with the appearance of dilated cardiomyopathy seen in only a small percentage. The appearance of the end stage can vary – it can be of rapid onset, accelerated progression, or a slow process – and this may manifest at any age.

STRAIN IMAGING

Speckle tracking echocardiography, a recently introduced specialized application and a validated method that is not angle-dependent, is now widely used in routine echocardiography to measure myocardial deformation or strain as a measure of LV systolic function [30]. It can provide measurements of both regional and global functions of the LV and the RV and LA chambers. This unique ability of STE provides a way to identify regional areas of myocardial dysfunction (due to fibrosis), seen as low segmental strain and paradoxical systolic stretch (Figure 4.20). Many studies have described a good correlation between reduced strain and myocardial fibrosis. The parametric strain image (bull's eye) can differentiate to some extent the LVH of hypertensive heart disease with that of HCM, with its striking involvement of reduced strain in the septum being indicative of HCM.

The parameters of longitudinal, circumferential (Figure 4.21), and radial strain provides incremental information over and beyond LVEF when assessing LV systolic function, especially in the presence of normal LVEF. Global longitudinal strain (GLS) has established itself as a sensitive measure of myocardial function compared to 2D-LVEF [31]. The presence of reduced GLS

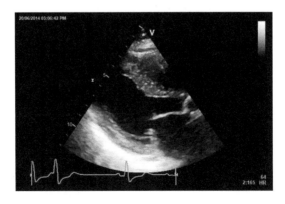

Figure 4.19 Dilated and dysfunctional LV of end-stage HCM. Note the preserved thickness of the septum, despite the end phase.

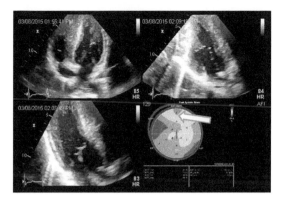

Figure 4.20 Speckle tracking echocardiography of the three apical views of the LV with decreased longitudinal strain. From the "bull's eye" parametric image, note the anteroseptum showing increased changes (pale pink segments) with paradoxical lengthening in the basal septum (blue segment) denoted by the white arrow, characteristic of HCM.

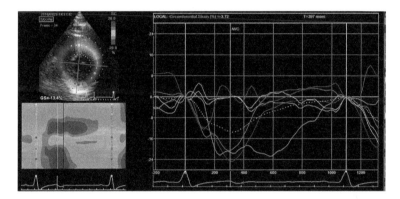

Figure 4.21 Speckle tracking echocardiography of parasternal short axis of the mid-left ventricle showing decreased global circumferential strain (white dotted line). Also, note the dyssynchronous segments (colored lines).

(less than 15–17%) is an early indicator of subclinical myocardial dysfunction even as the measured LVEF is seen to be within normal limits, demonstrating that GLS is more sensitive than LVEF in the assessment of LV systolic function. A compensatory increase usually follows the decline of GLS in circumferential strain. Recent studies show STE as a marker of future events, specifically a reduced LV-GLS with potential as a predictor of adverse cardiac outcomes in HCM patients [32]. It has also provided some insights into inter- and intraventricular dyssynchrony of LV, which is relatively common in HCM. Studies have shown that dyssynchrony is increased in HCM when compared to LVH of hypertensive heart disease. All parameters of strain are reduced in HCM compared to an athlete's heart. Speckle tracking echocardiography strain is not reliable when the 2DE images are suboptimal and proper techniques in acquisition and analysis are not followed.

DIASTOLIC FUNCTION
Most HCM patients have LV diastolic dysfunction with varying severity as the disease progresses. Diastolic dysfunction can be the earliest feature of HCM in some patients [9, 33]. The abnormal or thickened myocardium leads to impaired LV chamber compliance and stiffness, which results in varying degrees of diastolic dysfunction (Figure 4.22). The presence of a

(A) (B) (C)

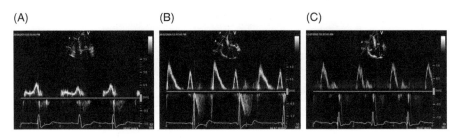

Figure 4.22   LV diastolic dysfunction of varying severity in different patients. (A) Grade 1. (B) Grade 2. (C) Grade 3.

restrictive pattern indicates an increased risk of adverse events. A small subgroup of patients who present with refractory symptoms that can be attributed to diastolic dysfunction and increased LV filling pressures have a poor prognosis. When faced with a diagnostic challenge in the presence of LVH in athletes, it is seen that diastolic function is always abnormal in HCM, while in athlete's heart it is supernormal. A comprehensive LV diastolic assessment must be made in HCM patients [34]. Unfortunately, HCM as a disease poses multiple challenges in the echocardiographic assessment of diastolic function, and many a time can result in an inconclusive study.

Diastolic parameters commonly measured are e' by TDI, trans-mitral inflow E & A velocities by PWD, the E/e' ratio, the LA volume, and tricuspid regurgitation (TR) peak velocity [23]. Other parameters of diastolic function (pulmonary vein sampling and the mitral "A" duration measurement) are to be measured if routine parameters are found to be inconclusive or if incremental information is sought. An E/e' ratio of more than 14 (average of medial and lateral annulus) is indicative of increased LV filling pressure along with LA volume of more than 34 ml/m², a difference of more than 30 ms between pulmonary vein atrial reversal duration and trans-mitral "A" duration and a TR peak velocity of more than 2.8 m/s. These parameters are not reliable and not advisable if the severity of MR is moderate or greater.

Traditionally, LA size has been a linear measurement ascertained by 2DE as an antero-posterior diameter in the parasternal long-axis view. Increased LA size in HCM can be due to long-standing diastolic dysfunction or mitral insufficiency, or both. An LA size of more than 4.8 cm indicates an increased risk of atrial fibrillation and other adverse cardiac events. Over the last few decades, LA volume has emerged as superior to the linear technique when assessing LA and is a better predictor of major adverse cardiac events. It is measured in the apical views as per standard methods, provided the imaging windows are acceptable. Increased LA volume (more than 34 ml/m²) reflects chronicity and severity LV diastolic function (with an associated increase in LV filling pressure) due to long-standing HCM. Impaired LA relaxation and filling in HCM individuals have also been noted, indicating that myocardial involvement is not confined to LV alone.

TISSUE DOPPLER IMAGING

Tissue Doppler imaging (TDI) has been used not only in diastolic function assessment but also to assess the regional systolic function of LV [34] (Figure 4.23). In HCM individuals, especially younger patients, when TDI, sampled at either the medial or lateral mitral annulus in the apical view, shows lower normal values of peak systolic velocities, it is suggestive of myocardial dysfunction (a peak systolic velocity of < 4 cm/s is a predictor of adverse events) [9]. Tissue Doppler imaging has been shown to have decreased e' in genotype positive, but a negative phenotype in individuals, indicating impaired LV relaxation and abnormal LV diastolic function. It shows the potential for early detection of abnormalities of the myocardium in this interesting subset of HCM. A TDI peak systolic velocity of less than 9 cm/s suggests a pathological

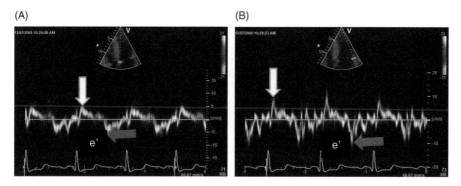

Figure 4.23 Tissue Doppler imaging of mitral annulus in the apical four-chamber view. (*A*) Borderline peak systolic velocity of septum (white arrow). (*B*) Normal peak systolic velocity of lateral wall (white arrow). e' denotes early diastolic velocity (red arrow).

LVH rather than a physiological LVH seen in athletes. TDI as a technique is limited by its application, because of its angle dependency and effects of cardiac translational motion.

CONTRAST ECHOCARDIOGRAPHY

Contrast echocardiography helps not just in identifying and confirming apical HCM, but also in differentiating it from LV apical aneurysm due to mid-cavity obstruction or non-compaction involving the LV apex. Contrast opacification of LV also helps in delineating an apically displaced PPM that can be mistaken for an apical HCM. The ability of 2DE is limited when it comes to identifying these conditions, but the use of contrast agents dramatically improves the imaging capabilities.

Contrast echocardiography has multiple roles to play in patients with HCM [9]. LV opacification helps to identify:

- Presence of LV apical HCM (also differentiates it from apical non-compaction);
- LV apical aneurysm in a mid-cavity obstruction (also detects the presence or absence of a thrombus);
- Enhanced endocardial border of LV, especially the anterolateral wall and distal segments which are not well delineated in suboptimal echocardiographic windows (LV opacification enables better visualization of the hypertrophied segments and also in assessing LV systolic function);
- The septal perforator branch for a septal ablation procedure (use of contrast has been shown to reduce ethanol quantity injected during the procedure and also reduces complications).

THREE-DIMENSIONAL ECHOCARDIOGRAPHY

Three-dimensional echocardiography, which is now part of mainstream routine echocardiography, offers incremental information by way of anatomical localization of abnormalities, identifying segments causing obstruction, and improving LVEF assessment of HCM patients [35]. There has been a gradual increase of 3DE over the years, but the advent of 3D TEE has accelerated its use in various situations, especially in interventions of the septum and MV. 3DE has been particularly useful in MV abnormalities: One such instance demonstrated that the medial structures of the MV are mainly involved in the mechanism of SAM and LVOTO. Other areas where 3DE is helpful are in the assessment of the LVOT area [36] during septal interventions of LVOTO (pre- and post-procedural measurement), measurement of LA volumes, calculation of LV mass, and for better visualization of apical abnormalities. The quality of 3DE images is affected by suboptimal echocardiography windows, while low temporal resolution leads to poor 3D images.

EXERCISE ECHOCARDIOGRAPHY

Exercise echocardiography is an alternative physiologic test to elicit potential gradients when other provocable methods are not possible or have been shown to be unsuccessful [9, 37]. An upright (not supine to avoid loading issues) bicycle or treadmill (Bruce protocol) exercise echocardiography is the preferred test to elicit latent/labile gradients, as it comes close to mimicking the physiological exertion that reproduces symptoms. This test is indicated in symptomatic patients, but whose resting peak gradient is less than 50 mm Hg [11, 38]. The appearance of a significant Doppler gradient on exercise is utilized for crucial clinical decisions, such as opting for interventions or medical management. Bicycle exercise has the advantage of obtaining better images. Limitations of exercise echocardiography are its inability at higher heart rates to separate the obstructive flow from an MR jet, which is a problem seen even on trans-thoracic echocardiography or TEE, but which is more difficult with exercise echocardiography. A hypercontractile LV may lead to a raised mid-cavity gradient, causing more confusion. Exercise echocardiography is also a predictor of future adverse events by way of the gradient elicited and also by way of the exercise duration the individual performs [39].

Dobutamine infusion (a graded increase up to 40 mcg/kg/min) and isoproterenol doses (up to 0.02 mcg/kg/min for 10 minutes) have been tried but are generally not ideal since they have a high rate of false positives. Dobutamine infusion is not preferred since the provoked gradients have low clinical value since they are not physiologic.

TRANSESOPHAGEAL ECHOCARDIOGRAPHY

Transesophageal echocardiography, a semi-invasive test, is indicated only in select situations [23]:

- Where inadequate windows on trans-thoracic echocardiography provide inconclusive images;
- Where cardiac magnetic resonance imaging cannot be performed due to technical or clinical reasons;
- For a better understanding of the mechanism of MR and LVOTO;
- For viewing MV anatomy (TEE provides excellent images of MV abnormalities, especially leaflet abnormalities);
- To guide interventions like surgical myectomy or septal ablation (pre-operative TEE evaluation is now a standard protocol before and after surgical myectomy);
- For detection of a ventricular septal defect or aortic regurgitation, post-myectomy;
- For providing morphological findings of coexisting aortic valve lesions or a suspected subaortic membrane [40];
- For the detection of direct insertion of anterior PPM into an AML;
- For atrial fibrillation patients in whom an LA thrombus is suspected or when cardioversion is planned.

1. Afonso LC, Bernal J, Bax JJ, Abraham TP. Echocardiography in hypertrophic cardiomyopathy: the role of conventional and emerging technologies. *JACC Cardiovasc Imaging.* 2008;1(6):787–800.

2. Rakowski H, Hoss S, Williams LK. Echocardiography in the diagnosis and management of hypertrophic cardiomyopathy. *Cardiol Clin.* 2019;37(1):11–26.

3. Elliott PM, Anastasakis A, et al. 2014 ESC guidelines on diagnosis and management of hypertrophic cardiomyopathy: the Task Force for the Diagnosis and Management of Hypertrophic Cardiomyopathy of the European Society of Cardiology (ESC). *Eur Heart J.* 2014;35(39):2733–2779.

4. Gersh BJ, Maron BJ, Bonow RO, et al. 2011 ACCF/AHA guideline for the diagnosis and treatment of hypertrophic cardiomyopathy: a report of the American College of Cardiology Foundation/American Heart Association Task Force on Practice Guidelines. *J Am Coll Cardiol.* 2011;58(25):e212–e260.

5. JCS Joint Working Group. Guidelines for diagnosis and treatment of patients with hypertrophic cardiomyopathy (JCS 2012) – digest version. *Circ J.* 2016;80(3):753–774.

6. Semsarian C, CSANZ Cardiovascular Genetics Working Group. Guidelines for the diagnosis and management of hypertrophic cardiomyopathy. *Heart Lung Circ.* 2007;16(1):16–18.

7. Smith N, Steeds R, Masani N, et al. A systematic approach to echocardiography in hypertrophic cardiomyopathy: a guideline protocol from the British Society of Echocardiography. *Echo Res Pract.* 2015;2(1):G1–G7.

8. Parato VM, Antoncecchi V, Sozzi F, et al. Echocardiographic diagnosis of the different phenotypes of hypertrophic cardiomyopathy. *Cardiovasc Ultrasound.* 2016;14(1):30.

9. Naidu SS, ed. *Hypertrophic cardiomyopathy.* 2nd ed. Cham, Switzerland. Springer Nature. 2019.

10. Losi MA, Nistri S, Galderisi M, et al. Echocardiography in patients with hypertrophic cardiomyopathy: usefulness of old and new techniques in the diagnosis and pathophysiological assessment. *Cardiovasc Ultrasound.* 2010;8:7.

11. Maron BJ. *Diagnosis and management of hypertrophic cardiomyopathy.* Massachusetts, USA. Futura, Blackwell Publishing, Inc. 2004.

12. Maron MS, Rowin EJ, Maron BJ. How to image hypertrophic cardiomyopathy. *Circ Cardiovasc Imaging.* 2017;10(7):e005372.

13. Rowin EJ, Maron BJ, Maron MS. The hypertrophic cardiomyopathy phenotype viewed through the prism of multimodality imaging: clinical and etiologic implications. *JACC Cardiovasc Imaging.* 2019;S1936-878X(19)30947-7.

14. Maron BJ, Ho CY. Hypertrophic cardiomyopathy without hypertrophy: an emerging pre-clinical subgroup composed of genetically affected family members. *JACC Cardiovasc Imaging.* 2009;2(1):65–68.

15. Maron BJ, Maron MS. Hypertrophic cardiomyopathy. *Lancet.* 2013;381(9862):242–255.

16. Hughes RK, Knott KD, Malcolmson J, et al. Apical hypertrophic cardiomyopathy: the variant less known. *J Am Heart Assoc.* 2020;9(5):e015294.

17. Hughes RK, Knott KD, Malcolmson J, et al. Advanced imaging insights in apical hypertrophic cardiomyopathy. *JACC Cardiovasc Imaging.* 2020;13(2 Pt 2):624–630.

18. Maron MS, Hauser TH, Dubrow E, et al. Right ventricular involvement in hypertrophic cardiomyopathy. *Am J Cardiol.* 2007;100(8):1293–1298.

19. Krecki R, Lipiec P, Piotrowska-Kownacka D, et al. Predominant, severe right ventricular outflow tract obstruction in hypertrophic cardiomyopathy. *Circulation.* 2007;116(23):e551–e553.

20. Samad F, Harland DR, Girzadas M, Jan MF, Tajik AJ. Athlete's heart vs. apical hypertrophic cardiomyopathy: look again! *Eur Heart J Cardiovasc Imaging.* 2017;18(3):381.

21. Sherrid MV, Balaram S, Kim B, Axel L, Swistel DG. The mitral valve in obstructive hypertrophic cardiomyopathy: a test in context. *J Am Coll Cardiol.* 2016;67(15): 1846–1858.

22. Silbiger JJ. Abnormalities of the mitral apparatus in hypertrophic cardiomyopathy: echocardiographic, pathophysiologic, and surgical insights. *J Am Soc Echocardiogr.* 2016;29(7):622–639.

23. Haland TF, Edvardsen T. The role of echocardiography in management of hypertrophic cardiomyopathy. *J Echocardiogr.* 2019. doi:10.1007/s12574-019-00454-9.

24. Maron BJ, Maron MS. The remarkable 50 years of imaging in HCM and how it has changed diagnosis and management: from M-mode echocardiography to CMR. *JACC Cardiovasc Imaging.* 2016;9(7):858–872.

25. Panza JA, Petrone RK, Fananapazir L, Maron BJ. Utility of continuous wave Doppler echocardiography in the non-invasive assessment of left ventricular outflow tract pressure gradient in patients with hypertrophic cardiomyopathy. *J Am Coll Cardiol.* 1992;19(1):91–99.

26. Maron BJ, Harding AM, Spirito P, Roberts WC, Waller BF. Systolic anterior motion of the posterior mitral leaflet: a previously unrecognized cause of dynamic subaortic obstruction in patients with hypertrophic cardiomyopathy. *Circulation.* 1983;68(2):282–293.

27. Geske JB, Sorajja P, Ommen SR, Nishimura RA. Variability of left ventricular outflow tract gradient during cardiac catheterization in patients with hypertrophic cardiomyopathy. *JACC Cardiovasc Interv.* 2011;4(6):704–709.

28. Minami Y, Kajimoto K, Terajima Y, et al. Clinical implications of midventricular obstruction in patients with hypertrophic cardiomyopathy. *J Am Coll Cardiol.* 2011;57(23):2346–2355.

29. Osranek M, Agarwal A, Jamil Tajik A. David and Goliath: a clash of flows in apical hypertrophic cardiomyopathy. *Eur Heart J Cardiovasc Imaging.* 2014;15(11):1280.

30. Maron MS, Pandian NG. Risk stratification in hypertrophic cardiomyopathy: is two-dimensional echocardiographic strain ready for prime time? *J Am Soc Echocardiogr.* 2010;23(6):591–594.

31. Tower-Rader A, Mohananey D, To A, Lever HM, Popovic ZB, Desai MY. Prognostic value of global longitudinal strain in hypertrophic cardiomyopathy: a systematic review of existing literature. *JACC Cardiovasc Imaging.* 2019;12(10):1930–1942.

32. Maron MS, Wells S. Myocardial strain in hypertrophic cardiomyopathy: a force worth pursuing? *JACC Cardiovasc Imaging.* 2019;12(10):1943–1945.

33. Nagueh SF, Mahmarian JJ. Non-invasive cardiac imaging in patients with hypertrophic cardiomyopathy. *J Am Coll Cardiol.* 2006;48(12):2410–2422.

34. Williams LK, Frenneaux MP, Steeds RP. Echocardiography in hypertrophic cardiomyopathy diagnosis, prognosis, and role in management. *Eur J Echocardiogr.* 2009;10(8):iii9–iii14.

35. Inciardi RM, Galderisi M, Nistri S, Santoro C, Cicoira M, Rossi A. Echocardiographic advances in hypertrophic cardiomyopathy: three-dimensional and strain imaging echocardiography. *Echocardiography.* 2018;35(5):716–726.

36. Pérez De Isla L, Zamorano J, Malangatana G, et al. Morphological determinants of subaortic stenosis in hypertrophic cardiomyopathy: insights from real-time 3-dimensional echocardiography. *J Am Soc Echocardiogr.* 2005;18(8):802–804.

37. Dimitrow PP, Cotrim C. Exercise echocardiography in hypertrophic cardiomyopathy. *Eur J Echocardiogr.* 2010;11(9):730–731.

38. Nishimura RA, Ommen SR. Hypertrophic cardiomyopathy: the search for obstruction. *Circulation.* 2006;114(21):2200–2202.

39. Rowin EJ, Maron BJ, Olivotto I, Maron MS. Role of exercise testing in hypertrophic cardiomyopathy. *JACC Cardiovasc Imaging.* 2017;10(11):1374–1386.

40. Kannappan M, Maron BJ, Rastegar H, Pandian NG, Maron MS, Rowin EJ. Underappreciated occurrence of discrete subaortic membranes producing left ventricular outflow obstruction in hypertrophic cardiomyopathy. *Echocardiography.* 2017;34(8):1247–1249.

Chapter 5

THE ROLE OF CARDIAC MAGNETIC RESONANCE IN HYPERTROPHIC CARDIOMYOPATHY

Gulhane Avanti, Lakhani Zeeshan, and Raj Vimal

CONTENTS

Cardiac magnetic resonance (CMR) has become a routine investigational tool for patients with hypertrophic cardiomyopathy (HCM), a notorious cause of sudden cardiac death (SCD) in the young, irrespective of symptomatology. Although trans-thoracic echocardiography (TTE) is the initial investigation of choice for HCM, CMR has to overcome its several limitations. It offers excellent spatial resolution with a capability to produce a striking contrast between the myocardium and moving blood, obviating the need for contrast adminstration and allowing visualization of those areas of hypertrophy not identified on echocardiography. Highly reproducible planning of the relevant cardiac planes allows accurate and reproducible assessment of ventricular function (ranging from hyperdynamic or systolic dysfunction) in HCM [1]. Cardiac magnetic resonance can assess the underlying etiology of clinical signs in HCM, such as exertional dyspnea due to mitral regurgitation, palpitations, and syncope due to arrhythmias related to interstitial fibrosis, chest pain due to microvascular dysfunction, and SCD due to dynamic left ventricular outflow tract obstruction (LVOT) obstruction [2]. Early identification of patients at high risk of major adverse cardiac events (MACE) and disease prognostication is possible with CMR as the presence and extent of myocardial fibrosis can be analyzed on late gadolinium enhancement (LGE) imaging [3, 4]. CMR can guide management strategies including consideration for primary prevention by implantable cardioverter-defibrillator therapy in patients with extensive fibrosis and thus an increased risk of sudden death by allowing scar quantification [5].

THE ROLE OF CARDIAC MAGNETIC RESONANCE IN THE DIAGNOSIS OF HCM

Cardiac magnetic resonance is recommended as a class I indication in patients with suspected HCM whose diagnosis cannot be cleared by echocardiography. In an adult, HCM is defined by a wall thickness ≥ 15 mm in one or more left ventricle (LV) myocardial segments – as measured by any imaging technique (TTE or computed tomography) or ≥ 13 mm in patients with a family history of HCM that is not explained solely by loading conditions [6]. In children, the diagnosis of HCM requires an LV wall thickness of more than two standard deviations greater than the predicted mean (z-score > 2), where a z-score is defined as the number of standard deviations from the population mean [7].

The diverse etiology for HCM necessitates a systematic search for the underlying cause of increased LV wall thickness. Several fatal inherited metabolic and neuromuscular diseases, chromosome abnormalities, and genetic syndromes, as well as non-genetic disorders such as transthyretin amyloidosis (TTR) and AL amyloidosis can mimic HCM. The chronic use of drugs such as anabolic steroids, tacrolimus, and hydroxychloroquine have been reported to cause mild LVH not exceeding a 15 mm wall thickness [8].

IMAGING FEATURES OF HCM ON CARDIAC MAGNETIC RESONANCE

Analysis of HCM on CMR includes morphologic assessment of the myocardium, its wall thickness, mitral valve and subvalvular apparatus, and papillary muscle abnormalities. Functional assessment is also made for diastolic and systolic function, systolic anterior motion of the mitral leaflet (SAM), LVOTO, LV cavity obliteration, and tissue characterization for identification/quantification of focal and diffuse myocardial fibrosis using LGE and T1 mapping sequences. The CMR acquisition protocol in HCM is tabulated as:

1 Scout images: In axial, sagital, and coronal body planes.

2 Anatomy: Free breathing T1W axial black blood imaging from diaphragm to above aortic arch with a slice thickness of 8–10 mm.

3 LV function: A cine balanced steady-state free precision (bSSFP) pulse sequence is used to acquire: a two-chamber (2ch), four-chamber (4ch), short-axis (SAX) stack from mitral valve to apex; LVOT in the horizontal and longitudinal planes with a slice thickness of 6–10 mm, an interslice gap of 0–4 mm, and a temporal resolution of ≤ 45 ms. The end-systolic volume (ESV), end-diastolic volume (EDV), the ejection fraction (EF), and LV myocardial mass is determined according to Simpson's rule.

4   Q flow: The phase contrast CMR is obtained through LVOT planes at the subvalvular, valvular, and supravalvular level, perpendicular to the direction of flow. Appropriate velocity encoding is chosen to prevent aliasing, and to identify peak velocity and pressure gradients. The spatial resolution is 4–6 pixels per vessel diameter.

5   Late gadolinium enhancement: 4ch, 2ch, and SAX stack images with an inplane resolution of < 2mm are acquired > 10 min after gadolinium injection (0.2 mmol/kg) and time to invert set to null myocardium. This is a segmented inversion recovery GRE sequence acquired during the diastolic period, with a read-out every other heart beat.

6   Parametric mapping: An appropriate vendor-recommened T1 mapping sequence (e.g., MOLLI), acquired pre- and post-Gd injection in short-axis plane at base, mid-, and apex. Post-contrast T1 maps are acquired after 15 mins of Gd injection. Hematocrit measurements are needed to assess the extracellular volume.

MORPHOLOGIC ASSESSMENT OF HCM
LEFT VENTRICULAR HYPERTROPHY

The most common phenotype of HCM is asymmetric septal hypertrophy, followed by mid-ventricular, apical, concentric, and mass-like subtypes (Figure 5.1) [9]. Cardiac magnetic resonance can identify segmental or diffuse areas of hypertrophy within LV, especially at the anterolateral free wall, apex, or posterior septum which cannot be reliably identified by 2D echocardiogram [10]. It can avoid overestimation of LV wall thickness when the crista supraventricularis, a right ventricular muscle structure, is situated adjacent to the ventricular septum and inappropriately included in the septal measurements on echocardiography [11]. Cardiac magnetic resonance offers excellent demonstration of LV apical aneurysms [12] and apical thrombi [13] and is more sensitive in the detection of subtle markers of HCM disease, such as hypertrabeculations and myocardial crypts [14]. Further, it is possible to perform genotype–phenotype analysis of HCM on CMR; patients with any genetic mutation are likely to demonstrate reverse curvature HCM in comparison to sigmoidal HCM or apical HCM (Figure 5.2) [15].

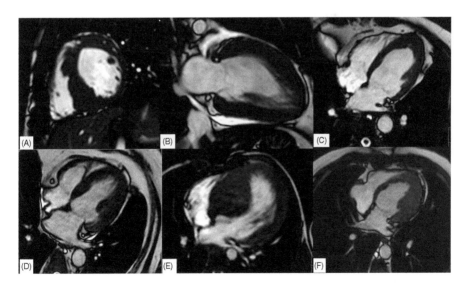

Figure 5.1   Different phenotypic expression of HCM depicted on CMR in various imaging planes. (*A*) Asymmetric septal HCM. (*B*) Concentric HCM. (*C*) Apical HCM. (*D*) Concentric HCM with associated RV hypertrophy. (*E*) Mass-forming HCM involving septum. (*F*) Mass-forming HCM involving LV lateral wall.

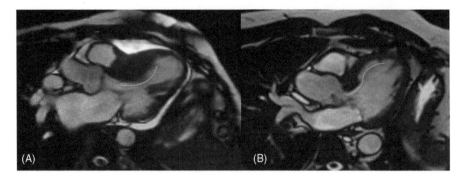

(A)   (B)

Figure 5.2   bSSFP 3ch view. (*A*) Patient with MYBPC3 mutation showing reverse curvature HCM. (*B*) Another patient with PKP2 mutation with suspected arrhythmogenic cardiomyopathy showing sigmoid curvature HCM.

MITRAL VALVE AND SUBVALVULAR APPARATUS

Mitral valve leaflet (MVL) abnormalities, such as elongation or accessory tissue, can be identfied on CMR in patients with HCM. It has been reported that MVLs are longer (27 mm vs. 21 mm in controls) in approximately 30% of patients with HCM. The MVL elongation can be > 2 standard deviations (std) above the length of controls [16]. In obstructive HCM, longer anterior leaflet measurements are observed with an average of 34 mm versus 24 mm in normal hearts [17]. Abnormal chordal attachment to anterior MVL and direct papillary muscle insertion into MVL can be seen in patients with sarcomeric mutations [18]. Although CMR also demonstrates mitral leaflet abnormalities, echocardiography remains the test of choice because of its superior temporal resolution and various Doppler techniques which provide hemodynamic information [2].

PAPILLARY MUSCLE ABNORMALITIES

Papillary muscle hypertrophy, accessory apical-basal muscle bundle, antero-apical papillary muscle displacement, double bifid morphology, and hypermobile muscles can be observed in many HCM patients with sarcomeric protein gene mutations [18, 19]. Papillary muscle hypertrophy is defined on CMR as papillary muscle thickness > 11 mm or greater than the LV free wall thickness. It has been reported that, in patients with HCM, papillary muscle mass can measure roughly twice the average mass in healthy counterparts and about > 2 std above normal with a cut-off of > 7 g/m^2; almost 20% of patients can demonstrate severe hypertrophy. Papillary muscle hypertrophy in HCM may not be caused by a primary genetic abnormality alone but could also be secondary to LV pressure overload from an LV obstruction. In addition, patients with HCM can also have multiple (i.e., three or four) papillary muscles [20]. Solitary papillary muscle hypertrophy is a unique phenotype of HCM that is seen in 19–20% of patients [21]. Anomalous insertion, accessory muscles, and anterior and apical displacement of the base of the papillary muscle is more common in patients with HCM than in healthy controls (77% vs. 17%) and usually involves the anterolateral muscle. This apical displacement of the base of the papillary muscle results in mitral leaflet slack with the mitral valve subsequently moving towards the septum, resulting in SAM and LVOT obstruction [22].

FUNCTIONAL ASSESSMENT OF HCM

Left Ventricular systolic function, either hyperdynamic or hypokinetic, can be accurately assessed on CMR using semi-automated functional assessment software. In early HCM, radial contractile function (EF or fractional shortening) is typically normal or increased, and myocardial longitudinal deformation is typically reduced at the site of hypertrophy [23]. Later, severe LV diastolic dysfunction is accompanied by marked atrial dilation with little or no LV dilation (the "restrictive" phenotype). As the disease progresses, a "burnt-out" or hypokinetic dilated phase can occur with a decline in LV diastolic and systolic function, mild-to-moderate LV dilation, and a fibrosis-related decline in LV wall thickness [24].

SYSTOLIC ANTERIOR MOTION OF THE MITRAL LEAFLET

The main advantage of CMR is in identifying the anatomy of the septal-systolic anterior motion contact and subvalvular apparatus in HCM on 3ch cine imaging. A widely accepted explanation of SAM is that raised flow velocities in LVOT, which is anatomically distorted by septal hypertrophy, creates a venturi effect, pulling the mitral valve leaflets towards the septum and obstructing the outflow tract [25]. However, studies with contradictory reports note that, at SAM onset, venturi forces which present in the outflow tract are of much smaller magnitude and that the pushing force of the flow is the dominant hydrodynamic force that causes SAM at normal LVOT velocity. Late diastolic and early systolic flow can strike the posterior surface of the protruding leaflets with a high angle of attack and push them into apposition with the septum. After mitral-septal contact, the pressure difference itself pushes the obstructing mitral leaflet further into the septum [26].

LEFT VENTRICULAR OUTFLOW TRACT OBSTRUCTION

In HCM, basal septal hypertrophy, SAM, papillary muscle abnormalites, and elongated mitral leaflets all contribute to left ventricular outflow tract obstruction (LVOTO) (Figure 5.3). Resting or provocable LVOTO is present in up to 70% of cases and is an important manifestation of HCM [27]. Dynamic LVOTO may also occur in other circumstances, such as calcification of the posterior mitral annulus, hypertension, hypovolemia, and hypercontractile states [6]. The identification of LVOTO is critical in the setting of drug-refractory severe symptoms since altered management strategies such as invasive septal reduction therapy with either surgical myectomy or alcohol septal ablation need to be considered in this patient subgroup [28]. Left ventricular outflow tract acceleration and flow turbulence can be diagnosed on CMR as a systolic signal void in flow-sensitive gradient echo (GRE) sequences. Peak velocity and the LVOT gradient can be quantified with phase contrast flow-sensitive sequences. Proper alignment of the CMR imaging plane is important to obtain the highest flow velocities as intravoxel dephasing and signal loss due to phase offset errors can make the accurate quantification of turbulent flow difficult with this technique [2]. An accurate marker for LVOT obstruction is the LVOT/aortic valve (LVOT/AO) diameter ratio as measured on CMR imaging compared to Doppler echocardiography [29]. An increased ratio of anterior leaflet length to the LVOT diameter on CMR is reportedly associated with resting and provocable obstruction [16].

LEFT VENTRICULAR CAVITY OBLITERATION

Apical and mid-cavity obstruction with associated apical aneurysms can be commonly noted in HCM (Figure 5.4). Apical HCM, also known as a Yamaguchi variant, is characterized by apical systolic obliteration and is associated with atrial fibrillation (AF), stroke, heart failure (HF), and mortality [30]. A double-chambered LV is rarely seen with an abnormal musculature/septum between the mitral valve and papillary muscles, dividing the LV into two chambers in HCM [19].

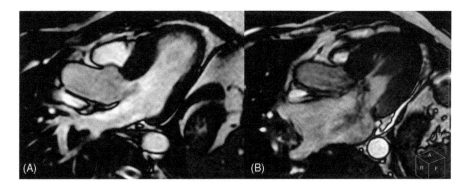

Figure 5.3 bSSFP 3ch view showing (*A*) mild LVOT narrowing in end-diastole and (*B*) basal septal hypertrophy and systolic anterior motion of mitral leaflet causing LVOT obstruction and mitral regurgitation depicted in end systole.

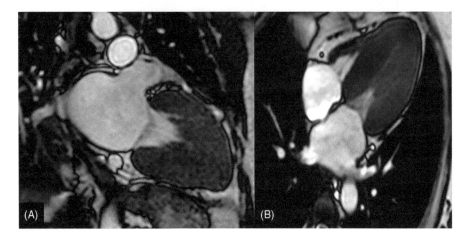

Figure 5.4   bSSFP 2ch (*A*) and 4ch views (*B*) showing LV cavity obliteration in two different patients.

MITRAL REGURGITATION AND LEFT ATRIAL ENLARGEMENT

Systolic anterior motion results in the failure of normal leaflet coaptation and mitral regurgitation, which is typically mid-to-late systolic and inferolaterally oriented with severity depending on the degree of the LVOT obstruction [31]. On CMR, the visualized regurgitant jet on a flow-sensitive GRE or bSSFP sequence can be quantified by subtracting the forward aortic flow, derived from the phase contrast sequence, from the LV stroke volume measured on cine images [32]. Left atrial (LA) enlargement occurs in most patients with LVOT obstruction, SAM-related mitral valve regurgitation, and LV diastolic dysfunction with elevated filling LV pressure. Left atrial size ≥ 45 mm is a consistent predictor for AF and stroke in patients with HCM, hence patients in sinus rhythm with an LA diameter ≥ 45 mm should undergo 6–12 monthly 48-hour ambulatory ECG monitoring to detect AF. The presence of atrial wall fibrosis detected on LGE-CMR serves as another important predictor of AF in patients with HCM [33].

DIASTOLIC DYSFUNCTION

This is a major contributor to the pathophysiology of HF in HCM, identified as a restrictive LV filling pattern with a ratio of mitral peak velocity of early filling (E) to mitral peak velocity of late filling (A) ≥ 2, and an E-wave deceleration time ≤ 150 ms on echocardiography [34]. Mitral inflow velocities and pulmonary vein flow can be derived from phase contrast CMR to assess diastolic dysfunction on CMR. Further, elevated LV filling pressure, transmitted in retrograde into the pulmonary circulation, leads to an increase in central transit time, pulmonary blood volume, and increased pulmonary capillary hydrostatic pressure, which can be measured on CMR to identify diastolic dysfunction in patients with HCM [35]. The pulmonary blood volume index (PBVI) measured by first-pass perfusion CMR imaging has been shown to differentiate between stages of diastolic dysfunction in patients with HF and a reduced LV ejection fraction, and has thus been proposed as a quantitative biomarker of hemodynamic congestion in HCM [36]. On CMR, the pulmonary transit time is defined by the time interval between the peaks of the two signal intensity/time curves for the right ventricle (RV) and LV respectively. Pulmonary blood volume index can be obtained as the product between the RV stroke volume index and the pulmonary transit time, normalized by the R-R interval. The best cut-off point of 413 mL/m^2 is a reported diagnostic of LV diastolic dysfunction, with increased left atrial pressure, with a good diagnostic accuracy [37].

TISSUE CHARACTERIZATION OF MYOCARDIAL FIBROSIS
LATE GADOLINIUM ENHANCEMENT PATTERNS

Focal or diffuse myocardial fibrosis can be unveiled on LGE-CMR, and serves as the pathophysiological substrate for malignant ventricular arrhythmias in HCM. Late gadolinium

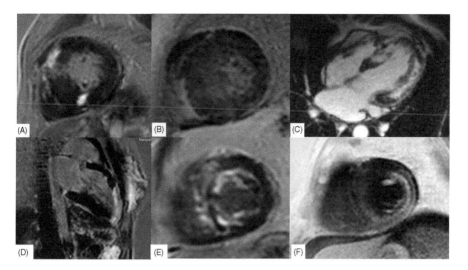

Figure 5.5 Late gadolinium enhancement with phase sensitive inversion recovery (LGE-PSIR) images showing different patterns of LGE encountered in different HCM patients. (*A*) SAX view showing RV insertion point LGE. (*B*) SAX view showing diffuse fibrosis in septum. (*C*) 4ch view showing mid-myocardial LGE in septum and lateral wall. (*D*) 2ch view showing transmural LGE in anterior wall. (*E*) SAX view showing mixed epicardial and subendocardial LGE in LV. (*F*) SAX showing papillary muscle LGE.

enhancement is present in the LV in almost 65% of patients, typically in a patchy mid-wall pattern in areas of hypertrophy and at the anterior and posterior RV insertion points (Figure 5.5). In the advanced stages of disease, full-thickness LGE in association with wall thinning is common [38]. Quantification of myocardial fibrosis on LGE is possible on CMR, but it varies substantially with the different methods employed, such as manual contouring, 2/3/5/6 std, and at full width at half-maximum technique (Figure 5.6); however, the 2-std technique is the only one validated against necropsy [39].

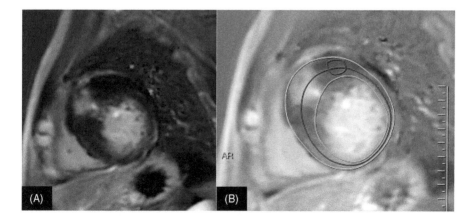

Figure 5.6 3D LGE-PSIR SAX view. (*A*) Shows focal fibrosis in basal anteroseptal segment. (*B*) Quantification of LGE percentage done using 6 std technique. The colored area has a computed LGE of 26% of myocardial volume in this patient with HCM. Note the small red circle in the anterior segment which is a region of interest drawn in a normally appearing myocardium for setting the pixel signal intensity value of a normal myocardium.

T1 MAPPING

Late gadolinium enhancement magnetic resonance imaging (LGE-MRI) can only delineate focal myocardial fibrosis but not diffuse interstitial fibrosis because the LGE technique defines the enhanced area based on the difference in the signal intensity relative to that of the normal myocardium; in diffuse fibrosis, a normal myocardium cannot be delineated on LGE. This issue has been addressed by myocardial native T1 mapping, an emerging non-invasive method to quantify diffuse myocardial fibrosis. Recent studies have shown that native (non-contrast) T1 mapping can differentiate the HCM myocardium from a healthy myocardium [40]. The native T1 value is prolonged in HCM and correlates with the wall thickness, suggesting that the former is a marker of the disease severity [40]. Left ventricular extracellular volume (ECV) can be calculated using pre- and post-T1 mapping and hematocrit assessment. A systematic review and meta-analysis of a multitude of studies show that native myocardial T1 values and ECVs are significantly increased in patients with HCM and dilated cardiomyopathy (DCM) compared with those in healthy controls, irrespective of the magnetic field strength of the scanner [41]. Extracellular volume can be used in the differential diagnosis of HCM vs. athletic remodeling in the hearts of athletes [42].

MYOCARDIAL OEDEMA IN T2 MAPPING

Myocardial oedema, as evident by hyperintensity in T2-weighted short-tau inversion recovery (STIR) or T2 mapping, is considered a marker of acute myocardial injury and may be noted in the presence or absence of myocardial LGE. In HCM, myocardial oedema may be related to chest pain, syncope, or increase in troponin T. The presence of hyperintensity on T2W CMR represents advanced disease, that is, a higher LV mass index, a lower ejection fraction and a greater LGE extent, an association with a higher arrhythmic risk score, and markers of arrhythmic burden (particularly non-sustained ventricular tachycardia [VT]) and autonomic impairment (decreased heart rate variability) [43]. High T2 values in T2 mapping is reportedly related to syncope in cases of asymmetrical HCM with higher T2 values (T2 ~61 ms) noted in these patients than the reference myocardium (T2 value ~47 ms) [44].

SEPTAL ABLATION: PREPROCEDURAL AND POSTPROCEDURAL IMAGING

Surgical myectomy (the Morrow procedure) is indicated in patients with an LVOT gradient $\geq$ 50 mm Hg, moderate-to-severe symptoms, and/or recurrent exertional syncope in spite of maximally tolerated drug therapy [28]. Specific abnormalities of the mitral valve and its support apparatus, identified on CMR, contributing to outflow tract obstruction, can help in adapting additional surgical approaches, such as plication, valvuloplasty, and papillary muscle relocation, and making myectomy more appropriate than alcohol septal ablation in some patients [28]. When there is a coexisting mid-cavity obstruction, the standard myectomy can be extended distally into the mid-ventricle around the base of the papillary muscles [45]. Selective injection of alcohol into a septal perforator artery (or sometimes other branches of the left anterior descending coronary artery) to create a localized septal scar has outcomes similar to surgery in terms of gradient reduction [46]. Cardiac magnetic resonance is extensively used to assess the effectiveness of alcohol septal ablation in terms of quantification of the amount of tissue necrosis induced, as well as the location of scarring and the regression of the LV mass following the procedure. Septal ablation may be less effective in patients with extensive septal scarring on CMR and in patients with very severe hypertrophy ($\geq$ 30 mm) [47].

Common diagnostic challenges and their imaging features on CMR [6] (see also Table 5.1):

1   The presentation in the late phase of the disease with a dilated and/or hypokinetic left ventricle and LV wall thinning.

2   Physiological hypertrophy caused by intense athletic training. The absence of fibrosis may be helpful in differentiating HCM from physiological adaptation in an athlete [11]. Additionally, CMR can evaluate other structural abnormalities frequently implicated in the sudden death of athletes, including arrhythmogenic right-ventricular cardiomyopathy and myocarditis [48]. CMR is well suited to comparing maximum LV wall

Table 5.1   Cardiac magnetic resonance features in conditions mimicking HCM [6, 85–89]

Differential diagnosis of HCM	CMR features
1. Mitochondrial diseases	1. Impaired LVEF, concentric LVH, and myocardial edema on T2-weighted imaging. Patients present with mitochondrial encephalomyopathy with lactic acidosis and stroke-like episodes (MELAS). 2. Characteristic pattern of diffuse intramural LGE in the LV inferolateral segments identified in patients suffering from chronic progressive external ophthalmoplegia and Kearns-Sayre syndrome. 3. Patients with MERRF and non-specific MM have no particular findings.
2. Glycogen storage disease (Danon/Pompe)	1. In Danon disease: concentric hypertrophy, subendocardial CMR rest perfusion deficits, and global subendocardial LGE. 2. In Pompe disease: normal LV and RV volumes, normal LV and RV ejection fraction, non-ischemic LGE in the basal inferolateral wall, and elevated global ECV values.
3. Lysosomal storage disease (Anderson–Fabry disease)	Concentric hypertrophy. Presence of inferolateral LGE. Native T1 values are significantly lower in patients with AFD compared with HCM and healthy volunteers. Pseudo-normalization of T1 values in the lateral-infero basal segment in patients with a focal fibrous scar visualized on the LGE sequences.
4. Infiltrative disease (AL and familial ATTR, wild type TTR [senile] amyloidosis)	Concentric hypertrophy, global/subendocardial or segmental LGE and a highly specific pattern of myocardial and blood-pool gadolinium kinetics caused by similar myocardial and blood T1 signals. Small pericardial effusion, thickening of the interatrial septum. Nodular thickening of the aortic valve, reduced left ventricular ejection fraction (LVEF). Grossly elevated T1 and ECV.
5. Malformation syndromes: Noonan syndrome	Biventricular hypertrophy and obstruction to the outflow of both ventricles.
6. Hypertensive cardiomyopathy	No RV hypertrophy, maximum wall thickness ≤ 15 mm, no diastolic dysfunction, regression of LVH over 6–12 months of tight systolic blood pressure control (< 130 mm Hg). LGE in the mid-myocardium and epicardium, but no LGE at RV insertion points or areas of maximal hypertrophy.

thickness before and after a period of systemic deconditioning. A regression of wall thickness by more than 2 mm supports a diagnosis of athlete's heart, while hypertrophy that remains present despite deconditioning supports a diagnosis of HCM [49]. Extracellular volume can also be used in the differential diagnosis of HCM vs. athletic remodeling in the hearts of athletes [42].

3   Patients with co-existent pathologies.

4   Isolated basal septal hypertrophy in the elderly.

5   HCM mimics: Concentric hypertrophy is more common in metabolic and infiltrative disorders. Biventricular hypertrophy and obstruction to the outflow of both ventricles is frequent in Noonan syndrome and associated disorders. Clues that suggest myocardial storage disease or infiltration include sparkling or granular myocardial texture, small pericardial effusion, thickening of the interatrial septum, nodular thickening of the aortic

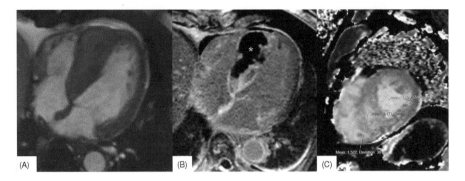

Figure 5.7 Patient with ATTR amyloidosis showing septal hypertrophy on a 4ch view bSSFP image (A) with area of hemorrhage (asterisk) and subendocardial basal LGE on an LGE-PSIR image (B). Native T1 map (C) showing raised T1 value reaching the blood pool, thus confirming intramyocardial hemorrhage on CMR.

valve, and mildly reduced EF with restrictive physiology. Anderson–Fabry disease is characterized by a reduction in the myocardial native T1 signal and the presence of infer-olateral LGE [50, 51]. Cardiac amyloidosis often shows global, subendocardial, or seg-mental LGE and a highly specific pattern of myocardial and blood-pool gadolinium kinetics caused by identical myocardial and blood T1 signals (Figure 5.7) [52].

PROGNOSTICATION OF HCM IN CARDIAC MAGNETIC RESONANCE

The estimation of SCD risk is an integral part of clinical management in HCM. Cardiac magnetic resonance is indicated for risk assessment in patients with a poor echo window, as well as routine assessment by clinical and family history, 48-hour ambulatory ECG, TTE, and a symptom-limited exercise test. Clinical features that comprise high risk for SCD include young-age, non-sustained VT, maximum LV wall thickness of ≥ 30 mm, a family history of SCD at young age, a left atrial diameter of ≥ 45 mm, LVOT obstruction, and abnormal exercise blood pressure response [28]. An apical cavity obliteration length of more than half of LV cav-ity height can predict the occurrence of adverse events in apical HCM [30]. Myocardial fibrosis (determined by LGE-CMR), LV apical aneurysms, and the inheritance of multiple sarcomere protein gene mutations can be used to guide intracardiac defibrillator (ICD) therapy in indi-viduals who are at an intermediate risk of SCD [12, 53, 54]. Cardiac magnetic resonance may be considered every five years in clinically stable patients, or every two to three years in patients with progressive disease as a class IIb recommendation for routine follow-up of patients with HCM [6]. An international multicenter Hypertrophic Cardiomyopathy Registry (HCMR) study has reported that CMR, or alternatively contrast echocardiography, should be performed for reliable identification of HCM patients with massive LV hypertrophy of > 30 mm, LV apical aneurysm, and quantification of LGE to identify a high-risk subgroup [55]. Cardiac magnetic resonance can guide prognostication of HCM patients in the context of the following.

EXTENT OF LATE GADOLINIUM ENHANCEMENT
Identifying those patients with HCM, in whom the risk of sudden death justifies the implanta-tion of a cardioverter-defibrillator (ICD) in primary prevention, remains challenging. A rela-tionship exists between LGE and cardiovascular mortality, heart failure death, and all-cause death, and a trend towards an increased risk of SCD [53]. CMR excels in establishing the extent of myocardial fibrosis which carries the most important weightage in the prognosis of HCM patients. There is a proven relationship between LGE and ventricular arrhythmias from 24-hour

Holter electrocardiography (ECG) records [56]. Chan et al. established the management principle for LGE in HCM and sudden death risk stratification and reported that it is not the presence of LGE that is important, but rather the extent and distribution of LGE in the LV as expressed by the percentage of the LV mass. They studied the prognostic utility of LGE-MRI in 1,293 HCM patients and demonstrated that LGE of ≥ 15% of the LV mass was associated with a two-fold increase in the risk of an SCD event in patients otherwise considered to be at lower risk [57]. A meta-analysis of more than 3,000 patients with fibrosis of more than 15% in the myocardium doubled the risk of sudden death, ignoring all other parameters [58]. Also, the risk of development of heart failure is directly related to the amount of fibrosis [59]. The amount of LGE areas of signal intensity of ≥ 6 standard deviations from a normal myocardium is recently reported to outperform the HCM Risk-SCD score and the American College of Cardiology Foundation/American Heart Association (ACCF/AHA) algorithm in the identification of HCM patients at increased risk of SCD, and reclassifies a relevant proportion of patients [60].

RIGHT VENTRICULAR AND LEFT VENTRICULAR LONG-AXIS STRAIN RATIOS AND TRICUSPID ANNULAR PLANE SYSTOLIC EXERTION

Cardiac magnetic resonance standard imaging planes can be used to calculate RV and LV long-axis strain (LAS) ratios, the LV ejection fraction, and tricuspid annular plane systolic exertion (TAPSE) measurement and serve as indicators of adverse prognosis in HCM patients. Left and right ventricular LAS are found to have been associated with SCD and aborted SCD caused by ICD shock, and can be measured as a percentage change in length measured from the epicardial border of the LV up to the mid-point of the line connecting the mitral annulus and the tricuspid annulus respectively in either 2ch or 4ch views. Tricuspid annular plane systolic exertion is calculated as the distance of the tricuspid annulus from end diastole to end systole in a 4ch view. Right ventricular LAS has been reported to be an independent predictor of adverse prognosis in HCM in addition to LVEF and TAPSE [61].

MYOCARDIAL ISCHEMIA

Patients with HCM have a significantly prolonged myocardial transit time due to coronary microvascular dysfunction. The two CMR techniques that are currently used to assess coronary microvascular dysfunction (MVD) through myocardial perfusion reserve (MPR) are velocity encoded coronary sinus flow measurements (CSF-MPR) and semi-quantitative myocardial first-pass perfusion [62]. The presence of MVD is generally associated with an increased risk of adverse events such as rapid progression and decompensation of heart failure, severe MVD, ventricular arrhythmias, and/or appropriate ICD therapy, as well as mortality [63–65]. The CMR parameter of the myocardial transit time (MyoTT) may contribute to the appropriate diagnosis and subsequent monitoring of MVD (not only in HCM patients) in a simple and non-invasive way – without requiring exposure to ionizing radiation or use of a pharmacologic stress agent. The myocardial transit time (cut-off of 7.85 s for HCM) can be defined as the blood circulation time from the orifice of the coronary arteries to the pooling in the coronary sinus (CS), and accordingly measured as the temporal difference between the appearances of the CMR contrast agent in the aortic root and the CS reflecting the transit time of gadolinium in the myocardial microvasculature. Robust correlation is present between MyoTT and LV global longitudinal strain in HCM patients [66]. Cardiac magnetic resonance-based measurement of coronary flow reserve can be achieved by calculating the ratio of flows in the CS during rest and maximal vasodilator stress [67].

MYOCARDIAL METABOLISM

Areas of myocardial enhancement at LGE-MRI and reduction of the myocardial phosphocreatine (PCr)/ATP ratio in phosphorus magnetic resonance spectroscopy (31P-MRS) are reported in HCM and indicate areas of increased interstitial myocardial space with fibrosis and impairment of myocardial energy metabolism, respectively. Cardiac magnetic resonance spectroscopy with phosphorus-31 demonstrates an altered myocardial energy metabolic profile in HCM that has been reported to correlate with the severity of LGE and thus poor prognosis [68]. This is not available in routine practice and needs dedicated systems.

GENOTYPE–PHENOTYPE RELATIONSHIP IN HCM

Cardiac magnetic resonance can establish the genotype–phenotype relationship in patients with HCM. It has been reported that patients with MYBPC3 mutations are found to have impaired ventricular function and may be more prone to arrhythmic events. Patients with beta-myosin heavy chain (MYH7) mutations show a higher LV ejection fraction (average LVEF 68.8 vs. 59.1, p < 0.001) than those with cardiac myosin-binding protein-C (MYBPC3) mutations. Patients with MYBPC3 mutations are more likely to have left ventricular ejection fraction (LVEF) < 55% (average patients 29.7% vs. 4.9%, p = 0.005) or receive a defibrillator than those with MYH7 mutations (average 54.1% vs. 26.8%, p = 0.020) [69].

PROGNOSIS IN POST-SEPTAL ABLATION PATIENTS

In-hospital post-operative atrial fibrillation (POAF) has been indicated as a poorer clinical outcome after myectomy for obstructive HCM patients, similar to those with preoperative AF. Elevated left atrial volume has been shown to be independently related to POAF onset in HCM patients who underwent myectomy [70].

In 4D flow, a reduction in the turbulent kinetic energy peak (TKE) (from 21.02 to 8.74 J) by 58% after percutaneous transluminal septal myocardial ablation in HCM patients correlates closely to the pathophysiologic change of decreased LV mass and the LVOT pressure gradient, thus suggesting that 4D flow TKE can be used to assess the burden of the cardiac load in patients post-septal ablation [71].

RECENT ADVANCES IN CARDIAC MAGNETIC RESONANCE RELATED TO HCM

3D WHOLE HEART CARDIAC MAGNETIC RESONANCE

Whole heart CMR sequences can be acquired to identify unique anatomical features in HCM patients, such as the presence of a steep angle between the aortic root and the LV long axis compared with control subjects. The acuteness of this LV aortic root angle correlates with age and the observed LVOT gradient [2].

CARDIAC MAGNETIC RESONANCE FEATURE TRACKING STRAIN ANALYSIS

Left ventricular global longitudinal strain (GLS) is an established robust measure of LV systolic function and superior to two-dimensional LV ejection fraction measurement [72]. Regional longitudinal strain assessment shows higher variability of the measurements as compared with LV-GLS; hence strain analysis needs to be standardized in HCM patients [73]. Pagourelias et al. showed that impairment in segmental longitudinal strain was significantly associated with the magnitude of wall thickness, the location of the most thickened segments, and the type of underlying histological changes in patients with LV hypertrophy [74]. Aberrant apical myocardial deformation on strain analysis can distinguish a subclinical HCM heart from a normal control heart [75].

Since contractile abnormalities are present even when left ventricular wall thickness is normal, CMR feature tracking enables identification of myocardial dysfunction not only in participants with overt HCM , but also in carriers of sarcomere mutation without left ventricular hypertrophy [76]. Overlap between large areas of LGE and myocardial regions with significantly attenuated strain can help identify the impact of replacement fibrosis on regional deformation in HCM patients [77]. Global longitudinal strain on CMR can be used to discriminate between hypertensive heart disease and HCM [78]. It is associated with LV mass index, LV ejection fraction, global native T1, and LGE volume. The wide distribution of myocyte disarray in HCM patients, in areas of normal wall thickness (up to >20% of the myocardium), can be well identified on CMR strain measurements in HCM patients as opposed to the pathophysiological processes in hypertensive heart disease [79].

4D FLOW ANALYSIS

New CMR sequences under development might allow for the routine three-dimensional acquisition of the flow pattern and velocities not limited by imaging planes, real-time velocity encoding, as well as accurate measurement of turbulent jet velocities [80]. Alteration of 4D flow MRI can visualize complex helical LVOT 3D flow patterns and quantify LVOT obstruction in the presence of high velocity systolic outflow jets. There is potential for combined application of pre- and post-contrast T1 mapping and 4D flow MRI for the characterization of altered hemodynamics and myocardial ECV in patients with HCM [81].

Currently, exciting technologies, such as inline quantitative perfusion mapping of the myocardium, multiparametric tissue relaxometry, and tissue phase mapping, are being developed with potential benefit for management of patients with HCM [82]. Further techniques, such as computational flow dynamics [71], mono- and bidomain models of propagating electrical activity [83], and structure/diffusion tensors appraising myocardial microstructural dynamics, are under current research development [84].

In conclusion, CMR is a comprehensive assessment tool in patients with known or suspected HCM. CMR-derived myocardial morphological parameters allow ascertaining the diagnosis, differentiating it from other mimics, and also provides significant prognostic information and risk prediction for SCD.

REFERENCES

1. Maron MS, Rowin EJ, Maron BJ. How to image hypertrophic cardiomyopathy. *Circ Cardiovasc Imaging.* 2017;10(7).
2. To AC, Dhillon A, Desai MY. Cardiac magnetic resonance in hypertrophic cardiomyopathy. *JACC Cardiovasc Imaging.* 2011;4(10):1123–1137.
3. Riza Demir A, Celik O, Sevinc S, Uygur B, Kahraman S, Yilmaz E, et al. The relationship between myocardial fibrosis detected by cardiac magnetic resonance and Tp-e interval, 5-year sudden cardiac death risk score in hypertrophic cardiomyopathy patients. *Ann Noninvasive Electrocardiol.* 2019;24(5):e12672.
4. Rowin EJ, Maron MS. The role of cardiac MRI in the diagnosis and risk stratification of hypertrophic cardiomyopathy. *Arrhythm Electrophysiol Rev.* 2016;5(3):197–202.
5. O'Hanlon R, Grasso A, Roughton M, Moon JC, Clark S, Wage R, et al. Prognostic significance of myocardial fibrosis in hypertrophic cardiomyopathy. *J Am Coll Cardiol.* 2010;56(11):867–874.
6. Elliott PM, Anastasakis A, Borger MA, Borggrefe M, Cecchi F, et al. 2014 ESC guidelines on diagnosis and management of hypertrophic cardiomyopathy: the Task Force for the Diagnosis and Management of Hypertrophic Cardiomyopathy of the European Society of Cardiology (ESC). *Eur Heart J.* 2014;35(39):2733–2779.
7. Kampmann C, Wiethoff CM, Wenzel A, Stolz G, Betancor M, Wippermann CF, et al. Normal values of M mode echocardiographic measurements of more than 2000 healthy infants and children in central Europe. *Heart.* 2000;83(6):667–672.
8. Sumpter MD, Tatro LS, Stoecker WV, Rader RK. Evidence for risk of cardiomyopathy with hydroxychloroquine. *Lupus.* 2012;21(14):1594–1596.
9. Chun EJ, Choi SI, Jin KN, Kwag HJ, Kim YJ, Choi BW, et al. Hypertrophic cardiomyopathy: assessment with MR imaging and multidetector CT. *Radiographics.* 2010;30(5):1309–1328.
10. Moon JC, Fisher NG, McKenna WJ, Pennell DJ. Detection of apical hypertrophic cardiomyopathy by cardiovascular magnetic resonance in patients with non-diagnostic echocardiography. *Heart.* 2004;90(6):645–649.
11. Maron MS. Clinical utility of cardiovascular magnetic resonance in hypertrophic cardiomyopathy. *J Cardiovasc Magn Reson.* 2012;14:13.

12. Maron MS, Finley JJ, Bos JM, Hauser TH, Manning WJ, Haas TS, et al. Prevalence, clinical significance, and natural history of left ventricular apical aneurysms in hypertrophic cardiomyopathy. *Circulation.* 2008;118(15):1541–1549.

13. Weinsaft JW, Kim HW, Crowley AL, Klem I, Shenoy C, Van Assche L, et al. LV thrombus detection by routine echocardiography: insights into performance characteristics using delayed enhancement CMR. *JACC Cardiovasc Imaging.* 2011;4(7):702–712.

14. Brouwer WP, Germans T, Head MC, van der Velden J, Heymans MW, Christiaans I, et al. Multiple myocardial crypts on modified long-axis view are a specific finding in pre-hypertrophic HCM mutation carriers. *Eur Heart J Cardiovasc Imaging.* 2012;13(4):292–297.

15. Rubinshtein R, Glockner JF, Ommen SR, Araoz PA, Ackerman MJ, Sorajja P, et al. Characteristics and clinical significance of late gadolinium enhancement by contrast-enhanced magnetic resonance imaging in patients with hypertrophic cardiomyopathy. *Circ Heart Fail.* 2010;3(1):51–58.

16. Maron MS, Olivotto I, Harrigan C, Appelbaum E, Gibson CM, Lesser JR, et al. Mitral valve abnormalities identified by cardiovascular magnetic resonance represent a primary phenotypic expression of hypertrophic cardiomyopathy. *Circulation.* 2011;124(1):40–47.

17. Ro R, Halpern D, Sahn DJ, Homel P, Arabadjian M, Lopresto C, et al. Vector flow mapping in obstructive hypertrophic cardiomyopathy to assess the relationship of early systolic left ventricular flow and the mitral valve. *J Am Coll Cardiol.* 2014;64(19):1984–1995.

18. Urbano-Moral JA, Gutierrez-Garcia-Moreno L, Rodriguez-Palomares JF, Matabuena-Gomez-Limon J, Niella N, Maldonado G, et al. Structural abnormalities in hypertrophic cardiomyopathy beyond left ventricular hypertrophy by multimodality imaging evaluation. *Echocardiography.* 2019;36(7):1241–1252.

19. Rajiah P, Fulton NL, Bolen M. Magnetic resonance imaging of the papillary muscles of the left ventricle: normal anatomy, variants, and abnormalities. *Insights Imaging.* 2019;10(1):83.

20. Harrigan CJ, Appelbaum E, Maron BJ, Buros JL, Gibson CM, Lesser JR, et al. Significance of papillary muscle abnormalities identified by cardiovascular magnetic resonance in hypertrophic cardiomyopathy. *Am J Cardiol.* 2008;101(5):668–673.

21. Sung KT, Yun CH, Hou CJ, Hung CL. Solitary accessory and papillary muscle hypertrophy manifested as dynamic mid-wall obstruction and symptomatic heart failure: diagnostic feasibility by multi-modality imaging. *BMC Cardiovasc Disord.* 2014;14:34.

22. Kwon DH, Setser RM, Thamilarasan M, Popovic ZV, Smedira NG, Schoenhagen P, et al. Abnormal papillary muscle morphology is independently associated with increased left ventricular outflow tract obstruction in hypertrophic cardiomyopathy. *Heart.* 2008;94(10):1295–1301.

23. Urbano-Moral JA, Rowin EJ, Maron MS, Crean A, Pandian NG. Investigation of global and regional myocardial mechanics with 3-dimensional speckle tracking echocardiography and relations to hypertrophy and fibrosis in hypertrophic cardiomyopathy. *Circ Cardiovasc Imaging.* 2014;7(1):11–19.

24. Melacini P, Basso C, Angelini A, Calore C, Bobbo F, Tokajuk B, et al. Clinicopathological profiles of progressive heart failure in hypertrophic cardiomyopathy. *Eur Heart J.* 2010;31(17):2111–2123.

25. Maron MS, Olivotto I, Zenovich AG, Link MS, Pandian NG, Kuvin JT, et al. Hypertrophic cardiomyopathy is predominantly a disease of left ventricular outflow tract obstruction. *Circulation.* 2006;114(21):2232–2239.

26. Sherrid MV, Gunsburg DZ, Moldenhauer S, Pearle G. Systolic anterior motion begins at low left ventricular outflow tract velocity in obstructive hypertrophic cardiomyopathy. *J Am Coll Cardiol.* 2000;36(4):1344–1354.

27. Maron MS, Olivotto I, Betocchi S, Casey SA, Lesser JR, Losi MA, et al. Effect of left ventricular outflow tract obstruction on clinical outcome in hypertrophic cardiomyopathy. *N Engl J Med.* 2003;348(4):295–303.

28. Gersh BJ, Maron BJ, Bonow RO, Dearani JA, Fifer MA, Link MS, et al. 2011 ACCF/AHA guideline for the diagnosis and treatment of hypertrophic cardiomyopathy: executive summary–a report of the American College of Cardiology Foundation/American Heart Association Task Force on Practice Guidelines. *Circulation.* 2011;124(24):2761–2796.

29. Vogel-Claussen J, Santaularia Tomas M, Newatia A, Boyce D, Pinheiro A, Abraham R, et al. Cardiac MRI evaluation of hypertrophic cardiomyopathy: left ventricular outflow tract/aortic valve diameter ratio predicts severity of LVOT obstruction. *J Magn Reson Imaging.* 2012;36(3):598–603.

30. Kim H, Park JH, Won KB, Yoon HJ, Park HS, Cho YK, et al. Significance of apical cavity obliteration in apical hypertrophic cardiomyopathy. *Heart.* 2016;102(15):1215–1220.

31. Sherrid MV, Balaram S, Kim B, Axel L, Swistel DG. The mitral valve in obstructive hypertrophic cardiomyopathy: a test in context. *J Am Coll Cardiol.* 2016;67(15):1846–1858.

32. Hundley WG, Li HF, Willard JE, Landau C, Lange RA, Meshack BM, et al. Magnetic resonance imaging assessment of the severity of mitral regurgitation: comparison with invasive techniques. *Circulation.* 1995;92(5):1151–1158.

33. Guttmann OP, Rahman MS, O'Mahony C, Anastasakis A, Elliott PM. Atrial fibrillation and thromboembolism in patients with hypertrophic cardiomyopathy: systematic review. *Heart.* 2014;100(6):465–472.

34. Biagini E, Spirito P, Rocchi G, Ferlito M, Rosmini S, Lai F, et al. Prognostic implications of the Doppler restrictive filling pattern in hypertrophic cardiomyopathy. *Am J Cardiol.* 2009;104(12):1727–1731.

35. Cao JJ, Li L, McLaughlin J, Passick M. Prolonged central circulation transit time in patients with HFpEF and HFrEF by magnetic resonance imaging. *Eur Heart J Cardiovasc Imaging.* 2018;19(3):339–346.

36. Ricci F, Barison A, Todiere G, Mantini C, Cotroneo AR, Emdin M, et al. Prognostic value of pulmonary blood volume by first-pass contrast-enhanced CMR in heart failure outpatients: the PROVE-HF study. *Eur Heart J Cardiovasc Imaging.* 2018;19(8):896–904.

37. Ricci F, Aung N, Thomson R, Boubertakh R, Camaioni C, Doimo S, et al. Pulmonary blood volume index as a quantitative biomarker of haemodynamic congestion in hypertrophic cardiomyopathy. *Eur Heart J Cardiovasc Imaging.* 2019;20(12):1368–1376.

38. Rudolph A, Abdel-Aty H, Bohl S, Boye P, Zagrosek A, Dietz R, et al. Noninvasive detection of fibrosis applying contrast-enhanced cardiac magnetic resonance in different forms of left ventricular hypertrophy relation to remodeling. *J Am Coll Cardiol.* 2009;53(3):284–291.

39. Moon JC, Reed E, Sheppard MN, Elkington AG, Ho SY, Burke M, et al. The histologic basis of late gadolinium enhancement cardiovascular magnetic resonance in hypertrophic cardiomyopathy. *J Am Coll Cardiol.* 2004;43(12):2260–2264.

40. Puntmann VO, Voigt T, Chen Z, Mayr M, Karim R, Rhode K, et al. Native T1 mapping in differentiation of normal myocardium from diffuse disease in hypertrophic and dilated cardiomyopathy. *JACC Cardiovasc Imaging.* 2013;6(4):475–484.

41. Minegishi S, Kato S, Takase-Minegishi K, Horita N, Azushima K, Wakui H, et al. Native T1 time and extracellular volume fraction in differentiation of normal myocardium from non-ischemic dilated and hypertrophic cardiomyopathy myocardium: a systematic review and meta-analysis. *Int J Cardiol Heart Vasc.* 2019;25:100422.

42. Swoboda PP, McDiarmid AK, Erhayiem B, Broadbent DA, Dobson LE, Garg P, et al. Assessing myocardial extracellular volume by T1 mapping to distinguish hypertrophic cardiomyopathy from athlete's heart. *J Am Coll Cardiol.* 2016;67(18):2189–2190.

43. Todiere G, Pisciella L, Barison A, Del Franco A, Zachara E, Piaggi P, et al. Abnormal T2-STIR magnetic resonance in hypertrophic cardiomyopathy: a marker of advanced disease and electrical myocardial instability. *PLoS One.* 2014;9(10):e111366.

44. Amano Y, Aita K, Yamada F, Kitamura M, Kumita S. Distribution and clinical significance of high signal intensity of the myocardium on T2-weighted images in 2 phenotypes of hypertrophic cardiomyopathy. *J Comput Assist Tomogr.* 2015;39(6):951–955.

45. Dearani JA, Ommen SR, Gersh BJ, Schaff HV, Danielson GK. Surgery insight: septal myectomy for obstructive hypertrophic cardiomyopathy – the Mayo Clinic experience. *Nat Clin Pract Cardiovasc Med.* 2007;4(9):503–512.

46. Fernandes VL, Nielsen C, Nagueh SF, Herrin AE, Slifka C, Franklin J, et al. Follow-up of alcohol septal ablation for symptomatic hypertrophic obstructive cardiomyopathy: the Baylor and Medical University of South Carolina experience 1996 to 2007. *JACC Cardiovasc Interv.* 2008;1(5):561–570.

47. Valeti US, Nishimura RA, Holmes DR, Araoz PA, Glockner JF, Breen JF, et al. Comparison of surgical septal myectomy and alcohol septal ablation with cardiac magnetic resonance imaging in patients with hypertrophic obstructive cardiomyopathy. *J Am Coll Cardiol.* 2007;49(3):350–357.

48. Harmon KG, Asif IM, Maleszewski JJ, Owens DS, Prutkin JM, Salerno JC, et al. Incidence, cause, and comparative frequency of sudden cardiac death in National Collegiate Athletic Association Athletes: a decade in review. *Circulation.* 2015;132(1):10–19.

49. Caselli S, Maron MS, Urbano-Moral JA, Pandian NG, Maron BJ, Pelliccia A. Differentiating left ventricular hypertrophy in athletes from that in patients with hypertrophic cardiomyopathy. *Am J Cardiol.* 2014;114(9):1383–1389.

50. Moon JC, Sachdev B, Elkington AG, McKenna WJ, Mehta A, Pennell DJ, et al. Gadolinium enhanced cardiovascular magnetic resonance in Anderson-Fabry disease: evidence for a disease specific abnormality of the myocardial interstitium. *Eur Heart J.* 2003;24(23):2151–2155.

51. Sado DM, White SK, Piechnik SK, Banypersad SM, Treibel T, Captur G, et al. Identification and assessment of Anderson-Fabry disease by cardiovascular magnetic resonance non-contrast myocardial T1 mapping. *Circ Cardiovasc Imaging.* 2013;6(3):392–398.

52. Syed IS, Glockner JF, Feng D, Araoz PA, Martinez MW, Edwards WD, et al. Role of cardiac magnetic resonance imaging in the detection of cardiac amyloidosis. *JACC Cardiovasc Imaging.* 2010;3(2):155–164.

53. Green JJ, Berger JS, Kramer CM, Salerno M. Prognostic value of late gadolinium enhancement in clinical outcomes for hypertrophic cardiomyopathy. *JACC Cardiovasc Imaging.* 2012;5(4):370–377.

54. Ingles J, Doolan A, Chiu C, Seidman J, Seidman C, Semsarian C. Compound and double mutations in patients with hypertrophic cardiomyopathy: implications for genetic testing and counselling. *J Med Genet.* 2005;42(10):e59.

55. Kramer CM, Appelbaum E, Desai MY, Desvigne-Nickens P, DiMarco JP, Friedrich MG, et al. Hypertrophic cardiomyopathy registry: the rationale and design of an international, observational study of hypertrophic cardiomyopathy. *Am Heart J.* 2015;170(2):223–230.

56. Adabag AS, Maron BJ, Appelbaum E, Harrigan CJ, Buros JL, Gibson CM, et al. Occurrence and frequency of arrhythmias in hypertrophic cardiomyopathy in relation to delayed enhancement on cardiovascular magnetic resonance. *J Am Coll Cardiol.* 2008;51(14):1369–1374.

57. Chan RH, Maron BJ, Olivotto I, Pencina MJ, Assenza GE, Haas T, et al. Prognostic value of quantitative contrast-enhanced cardiovascular magnetic resonance for the evaluation of sudden death risk in patients with hypertrophic cardiomyopathy. *Circulation.* 2014;130(6):484–495.

58. Weng Z, Yao J, Chan RH, He J, Yang X, Zhou Y, et al. Prognostic value of LGE-CMR in HCM: a meta-analysis. *JACC Cardiovasc Imaging.* 2016;9(12):1392–1402.

59. Maron BJ, Maron MS. LGE means better selection of HCM patients for primary prevention implantable defibrillators. *JACC Cardiovasc Imaging.* 2016;9(12):1403–1406.

60. Freitas P, Ferreira AM, Arteaga-Fernández E, de Oliveira Antunes M, Mesquita J, Abecasis J, et al. The amount of late gadolinium enhancement outperforms current guideline-recommended criteria in the identification of patients with hypertrophic cardiomyopathy at risk of sudden cardiac death. *J Cardiovasc Magn Reson.* 2019;21(1):50.

61. Yang F, Wang J, Li Y, Li W, Xu Y, Wan K, et al. The prognostic value of biventricular long axis strain using standard cardiovascular magnetic resonance imaging in patients with hypertrophic cardiomyopathy. *Int J Cardiol.* 2019;294:43–49.

62. Bietenbeck M, Florian A, Shomanova Z, Meier C, Yilmaz A. Reduced global myocardial perfusion reserve in DCM and HCM patients assessed by CMR-based velocity-encoded coronary sinus flow measurements and first-pass perfusion imaging. *Clin Res Cardiol.* 2018;107(11):1062–1070.

63. Taqueti VR, Solomon SD, Shah AM, Desai AS, Groarke JD, Osborne MT, et al. Coronary microvascular dysfunction and future risk of heart failure with preserved ejection fraction. *Eur Heart J.* 2018;39(10):840–849.

64. Gould KL, Johnson NP. Coronary physiology beyond coronary flow reserve in microvascular angina: JACC state-of-the-art review. *J Am Coll Cardiol.* 2018;72(21):2642–2662.

65. Tower-Rader A, Mohananey D, To A, Lever HM, Popovic ZB, Desai MY. Prognostic value of global longitudinal strain in hypertrophic cardiomyopathy: a systematic review of existing literature. *JACC Cardiovasc Imaging.* 2019;12(10):1930–1942.

66. Chatzantonis G, Bietenbeck M, Florian A, Meier C, Korthals D, Reinecke H, et al. "Myocardial transit-time" (MyoTT): a novel and easy-to-perform CMR parameter to assess microvascular disease. *Clin Res Cardiol.* 2019. doi: 10.1007/s00392-020-01611-2.

67. Dandekar VK, Bauml MA, Ertel AW, Dickens C, Gonzalez RC, Farzaneh-Far A. Assessment of global myocardial perfusion reserve using cardiovascular magnetic resonance of coronary sinus flow at 3 Tesla. *J Cardiovasc Magn Reson.* 2014;16:24.

68. Esposito A, De Cobelli F, Perseghin G, Pieroni M, Belloni E, Mellone R, et al. Impaired left ventricular energy metabolism in patients with hypertrophic cardiomyopathy is related to the extension of fibrosis at delayed gadolinium-enhanced magnetic resonance imaging. *Heart.* 2009;95(3):228–233.

69. Miller RJH, Heidary S, Pavlovic A, Schlachter A, Dash R, Fleischmann D, et al. Defining genotype-phenotype relationships in patients with hypertrophic cardiomyopathy using cardiovascular magnetic resonance imaging. *PLoS One.* 2019;14(6):e0217612.

70. Tang B, Song Y, Cheng S, Cui H, Ji K, Zhao S, et al. In-hospital postoperative atrial fibrillation indicates a poorer clinical outcome after myectomy for obstructive hypertrophic cardiomyopathy. *Ann Thorac Cardiovasc Surg.* 2019;26(1):22–29.

71. Iwata K, Matsuda J, Imori Y, Sekine T, Takano H. Four-dimensional flow magnetic resonance imaging reveals the reduction in turbulent kinetic energy after percutaneous transluminal septal myocardial ablation in hypertrophic obstructive cardiomyopathy. *Eur Heart J.* 2019.

72. Barbier P, Mirea O, Cefalu C, Maltagliati A, Savioli G, Guglielmo M. Reliability and feasibility of longitudinal AFI global and segmental strain compared with 2D left ventricular volumes and ejection fraction: intra- and inter-operator, test-retest, and inter-cycle reproducibility. *Eur Heart J Cardiovasc Imaging.* 2015;16(6):642–652.

73. Delgado V, Ajmone Marsan N. Global and regional longitudinal strain assessment in hypertrophic cardiomyopathy. *Circ Cardiovasc Imaging.* 2019;12(8):e009586.

74. Pagourelias ED, Mirea O, Vovas G, Duchenne J, Michalski B, Van Cleemput J, et al. Relation of regional myocardial structure and function in hypertrophic cardiomyopathy and amyloidois: a combined two-dimensional speckle tracking and cardiovascular magnetic resonance analysis. *Eur Heart J Cardiovasc Imaging.* 2019;20(4):426–437.

75. Piras P, Torromeo C, Evangelista A, Esposito G, Nardinocchi P, Teresi L, et al. Noninvasive prediction of genotype positive-phenotype negative in hypertrophic cardiomyopathy by 3D modern shape analysis. *Exp Physiol.* 2019;104(11):1688–1700.

76. Vigneault DM, Yang E, Jensen PJ, Tee MW, Farhad H, Chu L, et al. Left ventricular strain is abnormal in preclinical and overt hypertrophic cardiomyopathy: cardiac MR feature tracking. *Radiology.* 2019;290(3):640–648.

77. Aletras AH, Tilak GS, Hsu LY, Arai AE. Heterogeneity of intramural function in hypertrophic cardiomyopathy: mechanistic insights from MRI late gadolinium enhancement and high-resolution displacement encoding with stimulated echoes strain maps. *Circ Cardiovasc Imaging*. 2011;4(4):425–434.

78. Neisius U, Myerson L, Fahmy AS, Nakamori S, El-Rewaidy H, Joshi G, et al. Cardiovascular magnetic resonance feature tracking strain analysis for discrimination between hypertensive heart disease and hypertrophic cardiomyopathy. *PLoS One*. 2019;14(8):e0221061.

79. Rodrigues JC, Rohan S, Ghosh Dastidar A, Harries I, Lawton CB, Ratcliffe LE, et al. Hypertensive heart disease versus hypertrophic cardiomyopathy: multi-parametric cardiovascular magnetic resonance discriminators when end-diastolic wall thickness >/= 15 mm. *Eur Radiol*. 2017;27(3):1125–1135.

80. Hope MD, Meadows AK, Hope TA, Ordovas KG, Saloner D, Reddy GP, et al. Clinical evaluation of aortic coarctation with 4D flow MR imaging. *J Magn Reson Imaging*. 2010;31(3):711–718.

81. van Ooij P, Allen BD, Contaldi C, Garcia J, Collins J, Carr J, et al. 4D flow MRI and T1-Mapping: Assessment of altered cardiac hemodynamics and extracellular volume fraction in hypertrophic cardiomyopathy. *J Magn Reson Imaging*. 2016;43(1):107–114.

82. Xue H, Brown LAE, Nielles-Vallespin S, Plein S, Kellman P. Automatic in-line quantitative myocardial perfusion mapping: processing algorithm and implementation. *Magn Reson Med*. 2020;83(2):712–730.

83. Pravdin SF, Dierckx H, Katsnelson LB, Solovyova O, Markhasin VS, Panfilov AV. Electrical wave propagation in an anisotropic model of the left ventricle based on analytical description of cardiac architecture. *PLoS One*. 2014;9(5):e93617.

84. Nielles-Vallespin S, Khalique Z, Ferreira PF, de Silva R, Scott AD, Kilner P, et al. Assessment of myocardial microstructural dynamics by in vivo diffusion tensor cardiac magnetic resonance. *J Am Coll Cardiol*. 2017;69(6):661–676.

85. Deborde E, Dubourg B, Bejar S, Brehin AC, Normant S, Michelin P, et al. Differentiation between Fabry disease and hypertrophic cardiomyopathy with cardiac T1 mapping. *Diagn Interv Imaging*. 2019;101(2):59–667.

86. Yilmaz A, Gdynia HJ, Ponfick M, Rosch S, Lindner A, Ludolph AC, et al. Cardiovascular magnetic resonance imaging (CMR) reveals characteristic pattern of myocardial damage in patients with mitochondrial myopathy. *Clin Res Cardiol*. 2012;101(4):255–261.

87. Florian A, Ludwig A, Stubbe-Drager B, Boentert M, Young P, Waltenberger J, et al. Characteristic cardiac phenotypes are detected by cardiovascular magnetic resonance in patients with different clinical phenotypes and genotypes of mitochondrial myopathy. *J Cardiovasc Magn Reson*. 2015;17:40.

88. Boentert M, Florian A, Drager B, Young P, Yilmaz A. Pattern and prognostic value of cardiac involvement in patients with late-onset pompe disease: a comprehensive cardiovascular magnetic resonance approach. *J Cardiovasc Magn Reson*. 2016;18(1):91.

89. Piotrowska-Kownacka D, Kownacki L, Kuch M, Walczak E, Kosieradzka A, Fidzianska A, et al. Cardiovascular magnetic resonance findings in a case of Danon disease. *J Cardiovasc Magn Reson*. 2009;11:12.

Chapter 6

SURGICAL STRATEGIES OF MYECTOMY FOR HYPERTROPHIC OBSTRUCTIVE CARDIOMYOPATHY

V. Rao Parachuri, Sreekar Balasundaram, and Ameya Kaskar

CONTENTS

INTRODUCTION

HISTORY OF SURGERY FOR HYPERTROPHIC OBSTRUCTIVE CARDIOMYOPATHY

Numerous techniques for surgical relief of the obstruction in hypertrophic obstructive cardiomyopathy (HOCM) have been described ever since Cleland [1] started with transaortic myotomy in 1958, a procedure which later on became better known as the Bigelow [2] technique. Septal myectomy rather than simple myotomy was introduced by Morrow [3] in 1961 and advanced over the years to the standard operation. It was based on the assumption that asymmetric septal hypertrophy was solely responsible for the left ventricular outflow tract obstruction.

Transaortic septal myectomy is currently considered to be the most appropriate surgical treatment for patients with HOCM with obstruction mainly confined to the left ventricular outflow tract (LVOT) which progresses with severe symptoms when unresponsive to medical therapy [3–20]. In patients with mid-ventricular obstruction and apical HCM, myectomy is performed through a ventriculotomy. However, there is a significantly steep learning curve for this procedure. Outcomes in the early surgical era were hindered by complications of complete heart block, ventricular septal defect, or injury to the aortic or mitral valves or both when resection was excessive or imprecise, while inadequate resection led to incomplete relief of obstruction and persistence of symptoms. Current surgical results are vastly improved, although the reported experience in the world is limited to a few tertiary referral centers.

Here, we discuss the various surgical techniques that we have employed for myectomy in HCM with LVOT obstruction, mid-ventricular obstruction, and apical HCM.

SURGICAL PLANNING OF MYECTOMY

Patient selection for HCM surgery is based on clinical presentation, risk factors and imaging studies. The main modalities of imaging are echocardiography and cardiac MRI. It is often productive if the surgeon spends time in the imaging department interacting directly with the imaging specialists so as to plan the extent of myectomy during surgery. A special note should be made of the extent of the septal thickening, in two planes: both circumferentially and longitudinally from the base to apex. Any additional locations of septal thickening at mid-ventricular and apical level should also be noted. Further attention should be directed to the right-ventricular side of the septum causing right-ventricular outflow obstruction which is vital and often ignored. These inferences can be immensely useful for planning the location and extent of incision along with the depth and extent of muscle resection. Additionally mitral and aortic valve abnormalities, such as a bicuspid aortic valve and the presence of anomalous muscle bundles, should be noted. The knowledge gained from personal discussion with the echocardiographer and radiologist will equip the surgeon with knowledge for adequate surgical pre-planning.

HYPERTROPHIC CARDIOMYOPATHY WITH LEFT VENTRICULAR OUTFLOW TRACT OBSTRUCTION

During surgery, the surgeon should utilize a good coaxial light system since most of the procedure is intra-cavitary with a limited field of vision (Video 6.1; https://www.routledge.com/9780367352813).

The strategy for cardiopulmonary bypass (CPB) used in our institution is single aortic and bicaval cannulation with tourniquets around both cannulae. This facilitates a bloodless field during surgery, while allowing any additional mitral valve surgery. Cardiopulmonary bypass is initiated by cooling the patient to 32 °C. At our institution, intermittent St. Thomas's blood cardioplegia is used for myocardial protection. The amount of cardioplegia used may be slightly more in HCM due to severe hypertrophy of the left ventricle.

A good exposure is the key for the success of this surgery. A near circumferential incision starting from the pulmonary artery on the left to just above the commisure between the left and non-coronary cusps gives the best view of the aortic annulus and LV cavity in our opinion (Figure 6.1(A)). Three 4'0' Ethibond sutures applied to the edges of the aortotomy facilitate the exposure of the aortic valve and subvalvular structures. Further exposure of the sub-annular area is done by passing 17 mm 4'0' Prolene sutures from inside the cuspal attachment, keeping it just under the annulus (Figure 6.1(B)). This is repeated for all the aortic cusps. These sutures safeguard the valve tissue against any inadvertent injury from the size 11 knife used to excise the muscle.

While performing an extended myectomy, we prefer a self-retaining malleable retractor blade placed under the junction of the right and non-coronary cusps for deeper exposure of the LVOT (Figure 6.2).

For protecting the mitral valve along with the chordae and papillary muscle we use the distal portion of the sump suction positioned across the mitral valve and the chordae to push it posteriorly and away from the line of excision of the muscle which is placed anteriorly (Figures 6.3 and 6.4). Alternatively a gauze can be placed inside the LV cavity in such a way as to push the anterior mitral leaflet and chordae posteriorly to avoid injuring the mitral apparatus (Figure 6.3).

The aortotomy free edge sutures and the aortic cusp retraction sutures are all fixed to the Frater suture organizer to give the optimal amount of traction (Figures 6.1 B and 6.2).

We utilize a gauze wrapped onto the sponge holding retractor for applying mild pressure externally over the sub-annular area so as to depress the anterior basal septum. This improves the exposure of the sub-annular septal myocardium and facilitates subsequent myectomy (Figure 6.2).

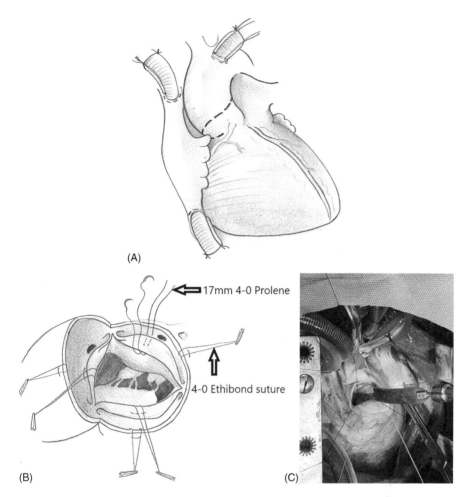

Figure 6.1 (*A*) The S-shaped incision in the LVOT extending to the non-coronary sinus. (*B*) Exposure of the sub-annular area by passing 17 mm 4'0' Prolene sutures from inside the cuspal attachment by keeping it just under the annulus. (*C*) The intra-operative picture is provided for better understanding.

Palpation of the heart should reveal the thickened septal area of the heart. Normally this thickening is felt anteriorly below the level of the aortic valve. Distinct thickened areas are felt in the mid-ventricular or apical regions respectively.

After exposing the sub-aortic valvular area as described above, the surgical plan for excision of the hypertrophic septum can be made. The location of the mitral apparatus, aortic cusps, and anomalous muscle bundles are noted. The circumferential excision is made in two blocks (Figures 6.2 and 6.5). Although this can be made as a single block we prefer to do it in two circumferential blocks. The first cut is made between two parallel incisions, one at the nadir of the right coronary cusp and the other at the level of the commissure between the left and right coronary cusps. The depth is normally about 1 cm unless the septal thickness is more than 2.5 cm, in which case the depth of cut can be 1.5 cm. All these measurements are arbitrary in that they are measured using an 11-blade cutting edge as a guide.

The initial extent of myectomy towards the apex of the LV cavity is about 2 cm. It is probably better to remove muscle in 1.5 cm circumferentially, 1 cm deep, and 2 cm towards the apex of the LV blocks than a single chunk, since the tip of the blade may drift too far into the septum, resulting

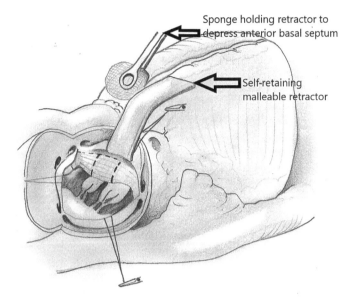

Sponge holding retractor to depress anterior basal septum

Self-retaining malleable retractor

Figure 6.2 Use of a self-retaining malleable retractor blade placed under the junction of the right and non-coronary cusps for deeper exposure of the LVOT.

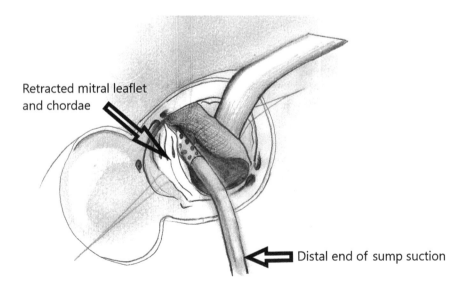

Retracted mitral leaflet and chordae

Distal end of sump suction

Figure 6.3 Mitral valve protection along with chordae and papillary muscle using the distal portion of the sump suction positioned across the mitral valve and the chordae and pushing them posteriorly and away from the line of excision of the muscle which is anterior.

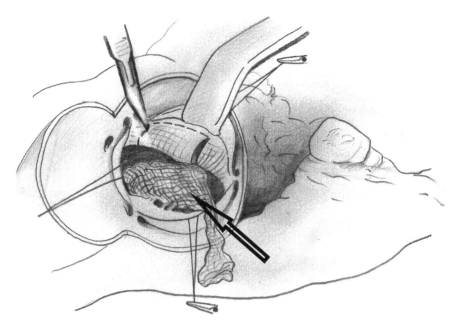

Figure 6.4 Mitral valve protection by using a gauze placed inside the left ventricular cavity in such a way as to push the anterior mitral leaflet and chordae posteriorly to avoid injuring the mitral apparatus.

in perforations in the LV free wall and septum. Also, blind deep incisions can injure the mitral apparatus. Following the initial circumferential block excision, the circumferential myectomy is completed by the second cut between the left fibrous trigone (left of the mitral apparatus) and extending clockwise into the previous incision (Figure 6.5). The amount of muscle taken out here should be not more than 0.5 cm since this portion of myocardium is rarely involved in the disease process and deeper incision can result in the free wall perforation at the left atrial appendage area.

Further myocardial blocks are excised to create a trench in the thickened septum towards the apex of the left ventricle, between the anterolateral and posteromedial papillary muscles (Figure 6.5). The trench thus created allows clear visualization of the papillary muscle origin and interior of the left ventricular apical area (Video 6.1; https://www.routledge.com/9780367352813). This is facilitated by placing the sponge on the stick and progressively compressing the ventricles from the outside. The trench should be directed towards the apex of the left ventricle and more towards the right side than the left side so as to avoid perforation of the free wall near the mid-ventricular level. Generally another one or two block excisions towards the apex should be sufficient. Sometimes hard fibrous areas are encountered while performing the trench and one is encouraged to cut a little deeper in these areas.

At the completion of the trenching both papillary muscles located laterally and posteriorly should be visualized well, along with the origin of these papillary muscles. It may be possible to visualize the interior of the left ventricle at this time.

As the resection proceeds deeper towards the apex, the width of the trench can be increased to 2.5 cm since the danger of causing damage to the bundle branch is much less. When the resection goes beyond the inferior edge of the septal thickening, further resection is stopped. This transition between the inferior edge of septal thickening and normal LV myocardium is indicated by appearance of LV trabeculae.

At this point, any loose muscles should be actively sought and excised. A thorough cleaning should be performed by the wall sucker to remove any muscle debris.

The aortic leaflets and mitral valve apparatus are checked at the end of the procedure to make sure no inadvertent damage has occurred to these structures.

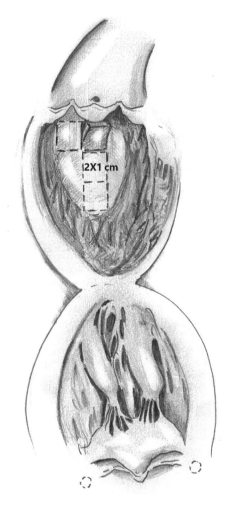

Figure 6.5 The circumferential excision is made in two blocks. The first cut is made between two parallel incisions, one at the nadir of the right coronary cusp and the other at the level of the commissure between the left and right coronary cusps. The second block is removed from the left fibrous trigone going clockwise joining the first block. The third block is excised from below the level of the first block. If needed the same process is repeted until the trabecular portion of the LV is seen.

The integrity of the ventricular septum is confirmed with the distended right ventricle by partially obstructing the venous return.

The aortotomy is closed in the usual manner either in two layers or a single layer using 4'0' Prolene suture. The heart is weaned off after complete rewarming and inserting two atrial and two ventricular pacing wires. At the time of weaning off CPB, inotropes should be used sparingly while avoiding vasodilators. All patients require cardiac output catheters as higher filling pressures have to be maintained throughout the initial post-operative period.

SURGERY FOR MID-VENTRICULAR HCM

Many surgical approaches have been described for mid-ventricular HCM. The one acceptable technique is described by Scaff and associates who use the fish-mouth incision at the apex of the heart. We modified this technique to make the incision 2.0 to 2.5 cm parallel to the distal left anterior descending artery (LAD) up to 2 cm above the apex in the anterior wall of the left

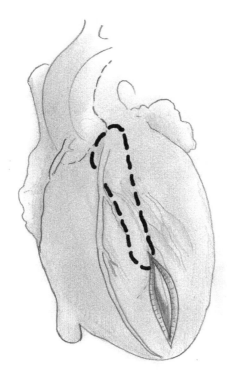

Figure 6.6 Myocardial blocks are excised to create a trench in the thickened septum towards the apex of left ventricle between the anterolateral and posteromedial papillary muscles.

ventricle (Figure 6.7). We believe this incision gives better visualization of the interior of the left ventricle. Also the hypertrophic septum is close to the incision and can be excised safely.

Four retraction sutures of pledgeted 2'0' Ethibond are placed partially within the thickness of the ventriculotomy. These are placed at the angles of incision and midway between the angles in order to effectively retract the edges of the incision. This also facilitates partial thinning of the muscle when the resection starts.

Planning the resection is based on a well-analyzed study of cardiac MRI and echocardiograms. The surgeon should have a good mental 3D plan of the myectomy based on these imaging modalities, mainly as to whether the hypertrophy involves the anterior or posterior interventricular septum. Generally, some LVOT resection as described above is required as it is our opinion that if only mid-ventricular resection is done, any associated mild LVOT obstruction may become pronounced. Therefore we prefer to do some LVOT resection through the aorta as described previously along with resection of the mid-ventricular portion through the apical left ventricular incision. The aim is to connect the trenches above from the aorta and below from the superior angle of the left ventricular incision (Figure 6.6).

Once the incision is made and the edges are retracted as described above, resection of the mid-portion is started. Generally the muscle in the superior angle is resected, maintaining a 1 cm thickness, a 2 cm width, and a 2 cm length directed towards the base of the heart. This avoids injury to the anterior papillary muscle base. At this stage, with the index finger inside and thumb outside, the thickened muscle is palpated. Inside, the LV cavity is examined for anomalous muscle bundles. If identified, these should be resected. With the initial resection the interior of the LV is better visualized. Next the path of interior resection depends on the location of the thickening. Generally the path for resection should be towards the lateral side of the aortic valve, extending towards the anterolateral commisure of the mitral valve. This avoids the

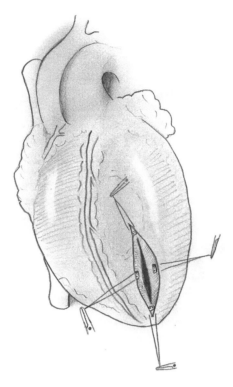

Figure 6.7 In mid-ventricular HCM the incision is 2.0 to 2.5 cm parallel to the distal LAD up to the apex in the anterior wall of the left ventricle.

conduction bundles. Sometimes the LVOT resection from above and the mid-ventricular resection from below can be joined together to form the continuous trench from the apical side of the ridge in the septum to the basal septum to below the lateral aortic annulus. Only 1.5 to 2 cm of trenching longitudinally should be done at a time to avoid cutting the papillary muscle bases (Figure 6.6). If these are cut inadvertently then they should be repaired using small pledgeted sutures. The chordae should be well protected. If these are injured, they are repaired through left ventriculotomy or through the left atrial approach. The chordae are repaired by commissural Alfieri or Gortex chords as the situation warrants.

Septal perforations are notoriously difficult to repair and therefore should be meticulously avoided, mainly by keeping the thickness of resection to 1 cm or even less towards the apex. Also avoidance of cutting the same site more than once should prevent this dreaded complication.

The most likely areas of septal hypertrophy are indicated by islands of fibrous tissue which are noted as one cuts the tissue.

Once the trenching is done across the hypertrophied tissue in the septum, the papillary muscles along with the chords are examined for injuries which are repaired as described. The presence of a ventricular septal defect (VSD) is checked by filling the right heart by partially clamping the venous line to note if any venous blood is coming out of the septum.

At the conclusion of resection the ventriculotomy is closed using a 1 cm wide Teflon (Bard soft), covering the entire length of the incision. Two layers of 3'0' Prolene with a 26 mm needle is used. A deeper multiple interrupted horizontal mattress suture, followed by a superficial over and over suturing technique is used for secure closure of the ventriculotomy.

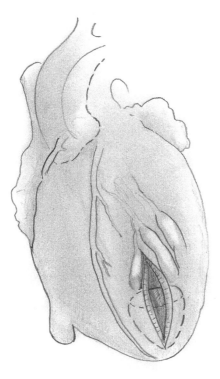

Figure 6.8 The surgical incision is the same as that described for mid-ventricular HCM except that the resection is extended more towards the apex.

SURGERY FOR HCM WITH APICAL HYPERTROPHY

This condition is rare in its isolated form. The surgical approach is the same as that described for the mid-ventricular except the resection is extended more towards the apex (Figure 6.8). Generally 0.5 to 1 cm tissue is taken from all around the apex including the lateral free wall and the septum. However, the septum is very thin near the apex so the thickness should be restricted to less than 0.5 cm. The aim is to increase the size of the cavity. Also the apical HCM may be associated with mid-ventricular and LVOT types. These should be dealt with as described earlier. Again care should be taken at the papillary muscle origin and septal level. Closure of the ventriculotomy is done using a Teflon support and two layers of 3'0' Prolene as described for mid-ventricular HCM.

WEANING OFF THE BYPASS AND ASSESSING THE ADEQUACY OF THE RESECTION

At the time of weaning, the usage of inotropes should be minimized. The CPB should be discontinued gently with higher filling pressures. After complete weaning, when the filling pressures are adequate, a transesophageal echocardiography (TEE) is performed to look for adequacy of the LV cavity and possible complications of the surgery. A 2D echocardiogram should reveal an adequate LVOT cavity and preferably the absence of systolic anterior motion of the anterior mitral leaflet (SAM), although some degree of chordal SAM is acceptable if the gradient across the LVOT is minimal (usually less than 20 mm Hg).

COMPLICATIONS OF SURGERY FOR HCM

Surgical resection can be fraught with many dangers, chief among which are ventricular septal defect and damage to the conduction tissue and the mitral apparatus, which includes the chordae, papillary muscles, and sometimes coronary artery injury. Aortic cusp injury and left ventricular free wall perforation can occur. The various complications and their respective management are described individually as follows (see also Figure 6.9).

CONDUCTION BUNDLE INJURY

This is a potential complication during myectomy. Conduction bundle injury can be avoided by planning the resection with due consideration. In general, keeping the line of resection to the left from the nadir of the right coronary annulus should avoid major damage to the conduction system.

AORTIC ANNULUS AND CUSP INJURY

Damage to the aortic cusp and annulus can occur from the knife edge during myectomy. Prevention of this complication is achieved by suture placement to retract the annulus as described above through all the three nadirs of the aortic annulus and by meticulously planning the initial incision. Also in the course of myectomy the knife needs to go in and out of the LVOT several times and each time attention should be paid as it traverses past the aortic cusps. Injury to the annulus can be repaired by figure of '8' interrupted 6'0' sutures. Occasionally a glutaraldehyde-treated autologous pericardium may be needed to augment the defect using 6'0' suture.

MITRAL APPARATUS DAMAGE

As the anterior leaflet is placed posteriorly in the aorta, it is vulnerable to damage from the tip of the knife during myectomy. The chordae along with the tips and belly of the papillary muscles, especially the anterolateral papillary muscle, are most vulnerable. Most damage to these structures can be prevented by paying attention and placing the sump sucker across the anterior leaflet and pushing it posteriorly during resection. Alternatively a gauge piece can be pushed into the LV cavity so as to keep the anterior leaflet and adjoining chordae, along with the anterolateral papillary muscle, pushed away posteriorly under the gauge.

Small papillary muscle tears can be left alone. Greater damage, which is due to inadvertent incision of the papillary muscle occupying a quarter of the circumference, needs to be addressed

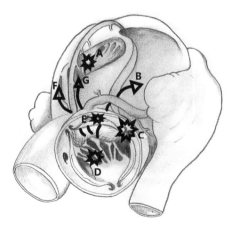

Figure 6.9 Surgical complications are mainly ventricular septal defect and damage to the conduction tissue and the mitral apparatus, which includes the chordae, papillary muscles, and sometimes coronary artery injury. Aortic cusp injury and left ventricular free wall perforation are potentially lethal complications.

with either 5 or 6'0' Prolene supported pericardial pledgets. Generally one or two sutures are enough for repair, which can be accomplished through the aortotomy, occasionally requiring an additional left atrial approach.

Chordal damage requires a strategy based on whether the commissural chordate or free margin chordae are affected. If commissural chordae are injured the commisuroplasty becomes a simple solution. On the other hand if the free margin chordae are involved, a neo-chordae using 4'0' Gortex chordae can be considered. An Alfieri stitch may be needed if free margin chordae, located centrally, are injured, wherein pledgeted 5'0' Prolene is used. Generally no annuloplasty is required as it may accentuate the SAM of the anterior mitral leaflet.

VENTRICULAR SEPTAL RUPTURE

During resection of the septum, this is perhaps the most dreaded complication. By adopting the aforementioned precautions this complication can be eliminated. The most important precaution is to keep the depth of resection not more than 1 to 1.5 cm, depending on the initial thickness of the septum as measured from the intra-operative echo. Also, one should not try to make a deeper excision at the same site. Another word of caution is that, as the trench is extended towards the apex, the next level of hypertrophic muscle should be identified before incision is made. Therefore, the prerequisite to avoiding septal perforation is that the trenching process should be done with uniform depth.

In the event of a VSD it is difficult to suture a patch either directly or away from the site, owing to the poor suture-holding property of the fragile muscle. It may be better to use a device placed directly or a surgically created device using a Gortex graft sutured to a large Gortex patch on both sides (personal communication, Dr Devi Shetty, Narayana Hrudayalaya, Bangalore, India).

Free wall ventricular perforations can occur when resection is done deeply into the left side of the LVOT. It may be located in the anterior LV free wall or laterally near the appendage. The LAD and left circumflex artery (LCX) vessels also may be injured in these areas. Patching with Dacron Vascular graft material (Haemashield) with multiple Teflon buttressed 3'0' Prolene is a better way to address this, rather than by direct closure. Low cardiac output following left ventriculotomy is rare due to the severe hypertrophy of the LV. Coronary injuries may need bypass grafting in addition to ligature of vessels at the site of injury and patch plasty.

POST-OPERATIVE MANAGEMENT

We advocate the routine use of a pulmonary artery catheter for all these patients. Excessive inotropes should be avoided. Filling pressures should be maintained higher than normal. Noradrenaline may be utilized to prevent excessive fluid administration and subsequent hemo-dilution. Supra-ventricular arrhythmias are poorly tolerated and should be appropriately managed. Routine atrioventricular pacing may be required to augment higher ventricular filling.

KEY POINTS FOR A SPECIFIC AND SAFE MYECTOMY

1   Good exposure.
2   Protection of aortic leaflets.
3   Preventing damage to mitral apparatus by a combination of intracavitory gauze or sump sucker placed across the mitral anterior leaflet, chordae, and anterolateral papillary muscle.

4   Planning the depth of resection based on the extent of hypertrophy seen from TEE and Cardiac MRI.

5   Initial circumferential excision followed by trenching towards the LV apex between the anterolateral and posteromedial papillary muscles.

6   Making sure that the depth of myectomy does not exceed 1 cm.

7   Trenching should be sequential from base to apex. One should not repeatedly make excisions at the same location.

8   Once the lower end of the hypertrophic hump is excised, no further trenching is required.

9   The success of myectomy is assured once the papillary muscle origin and left ventricular apex are reasonably well visualized. Once LVOT resection is complete, any additional mid-ventricular HCM should be addressed with a separate direct ventriculotomy incision at the lower one-third of the LAD.

10   Digital palpation may be useful to guide the extension of resection.

OUR EXPERIENCE

In our institution we have operated on 240 patients with HCM from 2012 to 2019. Most of them were HCM with LVOT obstruction. The mid-ventricular phenotype was seen in 23 (9.58%) patients. The need for concomitant mitral valve repair was in 21 (8.75%) patients, while three (1.25%) patients needed mitral valve replacement.

All patients were in NYHA classes III to IV, and 89% of patients improved to NYHA classes I and II following surgery.

There were eight (3.33%) deaths; six patients died of low cardiac output, out of which one patient had a ventricular septal rupture and one had an LV free wall rupture. One patient died due to respiratory failure and sepsis, and one died of low cardiac output complicated by sepsis. Surgical morbidity was five, two patients had a ventricular septal rupture, two had a free wall rupture, and two had an aortic cuspal injury. All these were repaired surgically.

Most of our morbidity and mortality occurred during our initial experience. Since we implemented the protocol-based approach during surgery, paying attention to depth of incision and avoiding injury to surrounding structures, these rates fell to near-zero levels. For the last consecutive hundred cases we have had no mortality or morbidity. Diligent pre-operative planning and care needs to be taken while performing myectomy. If all the surgical steps detailed above are followed, an optimal myectomy can be ensured without complications arising from injury to surrounding structures.

REFERENCES

1. Cleland WP. The surgical management of obstructive cardiomyopathy. *J Cardiovasc Surg* 4:489–491, 1963
2. Bigelow WG, Trimble AS, Auger P, et al. The ventriculomyotomy operation for muscular subaortic stenosis: A reappraisal. *J Thorac Cardiovasc Surg* 52:514–524, 1966
3. McIntosh CL, Maron BJ. Current operative treatment of obstructive hypertrophic cardiomyopathy. *Circulation* 78:487–495, 1988
4. Mohr R, Schaff HV, Danielson GK, et al. The outcome of surgical treatment of hypertrophic obstructive cardiomyopathy: Experience over 15 years. *J Thorac Cardiovasc Surg* 97:666–674, 1989

5. Mohr R, Schaff HV, Puga FJ, et al. Results of operation for hypertrophic obstructive cardiomyopathy in children and adults less than 40 years of age. *Circulation* 80:191–196, 1989 (suppl 1)

6. Williams WG, Rebeyka IM. Surgical intervention and support for cardiomyopathies of childhood. *Prog Pediatr Cardiol* 1:61–71, 1992

7. Theodoro DA, Danielson GK, Feldt RH, Anderson BJ. Hypertrophic obstructive cardiomyopathy in pediatric patients: Results of surgical treatment. *J Thorac Cardiovasc Surg* 112:1589–1599, 1996

8. Schulte HD, Bircks WH, Loesse B, et al. Prognosis of patients with hypertrophic obstructive cardiomyopathy after transaortic myectomy. *J Thorac Cardiovasc Surg* 106:709–717, 1993

9. McCully RB, Nishimura RA, Tajik AJ, et al. Extent of clinical improvement after surgical treatment of hypertrophic obstructive cardiomyopathy. *Circulation* 94:467–471, 1996

10. Wigle ED, Rakowski H, Kimball BP, et al. Hypertrophic cardiomyopathy: Clinical spectrum and treatment. *Circulation* 92:1680–1692, 1995

11. Schulte HD, Borisov K, Gams E, et al. Management of symptomatic hypertrophic obstructive cardiomyopathy: Long-term results after surgical therapy. *J Thorac Cardiovasc Surg* 47:213–218, 1999

12. Robbins RC, Stinson EB. Long-term results of left ventricular myotomy and myectomy for obstructive hypertrophic cardiomyopathy. *J Thorac Cardivasc Surg* 111:586–594, 1996

13. Williams WG, Waggle ED, Rakowski H, et al. Results of surgery for hypertrophic obstructive cardiomyopathy. *Circulation* 76:V104–V108, 1987

14. Cohn LH, Trehan H, Collins JJ Jr. Long-term follow-up of patients undergoing myotomy/myectomy for obstructive hypertrophic cardiomyopathy. *Am J Cardiol* 70:657–660, 1992

15. Heric B, Lytle BW, Miller DP, et al. Surgical management of hypertrophic obstructive cardiomyopathy. Early and late results. *J Thorac Cardiovasc Surg* 110:195–206, 1995

16. McIntosh CL, Maron BJ, Cannon RO, III, et al. Initial results of combined anterior mitral leaflet plication and ventricular septal myotomy-myectomy for relief of left ventricular outflow tract obstruction in patients with hypertrophic cardiomyopathy. *Circulation* 86:II60–II67, 1992

17. Krajcer Z, Leachman RD, Cooley DA, et al. Septal myotomy-myectomy versus mitral valve replacement in hypertrophic cardiomyopathy: Ten-year follow-up in 185 patients. *Circulation* 80:I57–I64, 1989

18. Merrill WH, Friesinger GC, Graham TP Jr., et al. Long-lasting improvement after septal myectomy for hypertrophic obstructive cardiomyopathy: Experience over 15 years. *J Thorac Cardiovasc Surg* 97:666–674, 1989

19. Minakata K, Dearani JA, Nishimura RA, et al. Extended septal myectomy for hypertrophic obstructive cardiomyopathy with anomalous mitral papillary muscles or chordae. *J Thorac Cardiovasc Surg* 127: 481–489, 2004

20. Dearani JA, Danielson GK. Obstructive hypertrophic cardiomyopathy: Results of septal myectomy, in Maron BJ (ed.): *Diagnosis and Management of Hypertrophic Cardiomyopathy*. Elmsford, NY, Futura, 2004, 220–235.

Chapter 7

MITRAL VALVE PATHOLOGY IN HYPERTROPHIC CARDIOMYOPATHY
Implications for Surgical Repair

Kevin Hodges, Nicholas Smedira, and Per Wierup

CONTENTS

INTRODUCTION

Over the last three decades there has been an increased understanding of the mechanisms of systolic anterior motion (SAM) of the mitral valve in hypertrophic obstructive cardiomyopathy (HOCM). Likewise, several mitral valve abnormalities have been identified, which exist in HOCM and may be independent of the degree of septal hypertrophy. With this new knowledge, surgeons have expanded the toolbox for managing left ventricular outflow tract (LVOT) obstruction by septal myectomy alone to include several targeted mitral valve interventions.

MITRAL VALVE PATHOLOGY AND SYSTOLIC ANTERIOR MOTION OF THE MITRAL VALVE

Dynamic LVOT obstruction in HOCM results from SAM of the mitral valve. Historically, this phenomenon was attributed to the Venturi effect. However, improvements in echocardiographic and magnetic resonance imaging (MRI) techniques have led to a more complex understanding of the mechanism of SAM.

In a seminal 1987 study, Jiang and colleagues found that SAM begins *before* left ventricular ejection. This discovery fostered a new understanding of the mechanism of SAM, emphasizing the role of drag forces. According to this theory, anterior and inward displacement of the papillary muscles in HOCM results in chordal laxity and a leaflet coaptation point that is closer to the outflow tract. This, combined with leaflet elongation and cupping of the free edge, orients the leaflets upward into the outflow tract at the onset of systole. Ventricular ejection then drags the leaflets anteriorly, resulting in LVOT obstruction and mitral regurgitation [1].

This new mechanism was assessed *in vivo* by Levine and colleagues, who showed in a canine model, that anterior displacement of the papillary muscle induces SAM even in the absence of septal hypertrophy [2].

THE SPECTRUM OF MITRAL VALVE ABNORMALITIES

Over time, the spectrum of mitral valve abnormalities in HOCM has become more clearly defined. Klues and colleagues demonstrated echocardiographically that the mitral valve leaflet is increased, without significant increase in the annular area [3]. This is driven primarily by increased anterior leaflet length. Maron et al. later demonstrated that mitral leaflets are elongated independently of other HOCM-specific disease variables, suggesting that this is a primary phenotypic expression in a subset of patients with HOCM [4].

Further, a subset of HOCM patients have been found to have a congenital malformation, in which one or both papillary muscles insert directly into the anterior mitral leaflet [3]. These abnormal papillary muscles tether the leaflet in a more anterior position. Likewise, abnormal secondary chordae, which arise from papillary muscles or the septum, can insert at the base of the anterior leaflet and tether it in an anterior position [5].

Illustrating the hemodynamic importance of mitral valve abnormalities in HOCM, investigators from Cleveland Clinic analyzed echocardiogram and cine cardiac MRI data from patients with LVOT obstruction and mild septal hypertrophy (septal thickness ≤ 1.8 cm). Predictors of maximal LVOT gradient were basal septal thickness, bifid papillary muscle mobility, anterior mitral leaflet length, and abnormal chordal attachment to the base of the anterior mitral leaflet [5].

As awareness of the spectrum of mitral valve abnormalities in HOCM has grown, so has the armamentarium of surgical techniques to alleviate LVOT obstruction. Whereas once surgeons could offer only septal myectomy, there are now a number of techniques to target the multitude of mitral valve abnormalities that may predispose to LVOT obstruction.

IMPLICATIONS FOR SURGICAL REPAIR

SEPTAL MYECTOMY ALONE
Septal myectomy remains the gold standard for HOCM, even in the setting of associated mitral valve abnormalities (Figure 7.1). An analysis of the Society of Thoracic Surgeons' database from 2014 to 2017 showed that myectomy alone continues to be the dominant strategy, accounting for 66% of cases compared to 34% for septal myectomy with concomitant mitral valve surgery [6].

Some have argued that septal myectomy alone should be the procedure of choice for nearly all patients with HOCM, regardless of mitral valve morphology. Surgeons from the Mayo Clinic reported a series of 2,107 septal myectomies in which only 30 patients (2.1%) required a mitral valve intervention for LVOT obstruction in the absence of intrinsic mitral valve disease (i.e., mitral stenosis or degenerative mitral regurgitation). Of 1,830 patients who underwent isolated septal myectomy, the percentage of patients with ≥ 3+ MR decreased from 54.3 to 1.7% [7]. The same group also investigated the relationship of septal thickness with post-operative hemodynamic outcomes. They found that septal myectomy alone was effective in eliminating LVOT obstruction with very low complication rates, even in patients with septal thickness < 1.8 cm [8].

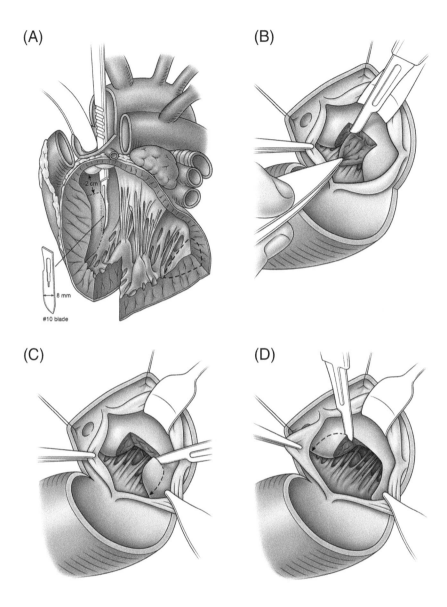

Figure 7.1 Extended septal myectomy is a three-step approach based on the location of the leaflet–septal contact identified on TEE. This contact is commonly 18 to 22 mm below the nadir of the right coronary cusp. Step 1: At this point, two parallel incisions are made 10 mm apart, 4 to 6 mm deep, and 15 to 20 mm long, with an inverted #10 blade (A). These incisions are connected using a #15 blade, and a rectangle of muscle 10-mm wide by 5-mm thick by 20-mm long is excised (B). Step 2: The edge of this excision is continued to the right trigone, removing another rectangle of muscle (C). Care must be taken to note the thickness of the inferoseptum in the four-chamber view, because it is often thinner than the anteroseptum seen on the long-axis view. Step 3: The anterior edge of the initial incision is then grasped and continued to the left trigone, removing another rectangle of muscle (D).

Opponents of this viewpoint would argue that, while isolated myectomy may suffice in most patients, adjunctive mitral interventions allow for a more modest myectomy and may increase safety in patients with limited hypertrophy [9]. This may be especially valuable for surgeons early on the learning curve.

The Mayo Clinic experience also demonstrates that there is a small subset of patients who require mitral valve interventions, even in the hands of an expert myectomy surgeon [6, 7]. Likely, these are patients with very abnormal mitral valve morphology or LVOT obstruction in the absence of significant hypertrophy.

TETHERING CHORDAE AND ANOMALOUS PAPILLARY MUSCLES

Patients with HOCM have been observed to have abnormal secondary chordae to the anterior mitral leaflet, which move the anterior leaflet into the LVOT and predispose to SAM. Often, these chordae are based in the septum itself, rather than the papillary muscle. Similarly, a small subset of patients have abnormal papillary muscles, which insert directly into the anterior leaflet [3] (Figure 7.2). Besides predisposing to SAM, these anomalies may produce fixed LVOT obstruction if the abnormal chords or papillary muscles are located within the LVOT itself.

Because they may contribute to fixed LVOT obstruction, it is our practice to resect abnormal secondary chordae or papillary muscles whenever these are present, independent of septal thickness or other mitral valve interventions [9]. In one small series of patients undergoing transaortic chordal cutting as an adjunct to limited myectomy, the combined procedure produced a more posteriorly positioned mitral valve position than myectomy alone [10].

ANTERIOR LEAFLET SHORTENING

Anterior leaflet elongation is an important contributor to SAM, which may occur independently of septal thickness. Intraoperatively, surgeons will observe an elongated tongue of leaflet tissue occurring at A2, associated with severely elongated primary chordae. Typically this segment is bounded on either side by normal primary chordae (Figure 7.3(A)).

Early in the Cleveland Clinic experience, A2 plication was the procedure of choice to shorten the anterior leaflet (Figure 7.3(B)). However, with continued observation that the elongated chords to A2 are nonfunctional, the authors have adopted the practice of a small resection of

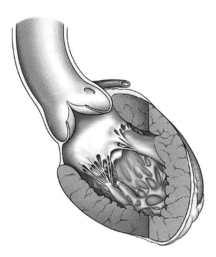

Figure 7.2 Tethering secondary chordae are often present on the anterior mitral leaflet that pull the leaflet into the LVOT. Resectioning these chordae allows the zone of coaptation to move posteriorly, away from the outflow tract.

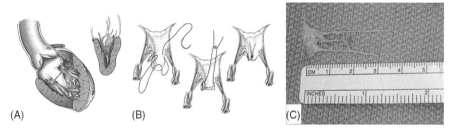

(A)   (B)   (C)

Figure 7.3   (A) Often in HOCM the A2 segment of the mitral valve is elongated, which predisposes to SAM. In this situation there are typically no normal chordae supporting the elongated segment. This segment can be plicated with a single stitch (B), or resected. (C) In this surgical specimen, note the excessively long and thin chordae attached to the A2 segment, which was completely resected along the dotted line shown in (A).

the redundant leaflet tissue by the free edge of A2, without additional plication or support with artificial chords (Figure 7.3(C)). In essentially all cases, the normal primary chords that border the resected segment are sufficient to support the anterior leaflet.

PAPILLARY MUSCLE REORIENTATION

The occurrence of symptomatic LVOT obstruction and anteriorly positioned, hypermobile papillary muscles without any septal hypertrophy led to the development of the papillary muscle reorientation operation. Early success in such patients led to broader application of this technique to patients with more significant septal hypertrophy [9, 11]. This has been replicated in several centers, suggesting that papillary muscle reorientation is an effective, reproducible technique for eliminating LVOT obstruction in appropriate patients [12].

Papillary muscle reorientation is performed through a transaortic approach, with or without concomitant myectomy. Abnormal, anteriorly positioned papillary muscle heads are identified, as well as corresponding posterior muscle heads that are fixed to the posterior left ventricular wall. Pledged sutures are used to fix the anterior muscle heads to their posterior counterparts to relocate them away from the outflow tract (Figure 7.4).

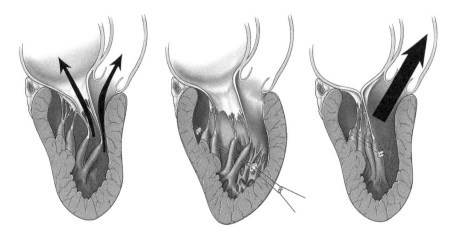

Figure 7.4   Large, excessively mobile or anteriorly displaced papillary muscles can contribute directly to LVOT obstruction and pull the anterior leaflet towards the outflow tract, potentiating SAM. Papillary muscle reorientation is performed by tacking anterior papillary muscle heads to posterior heads, moving the papillary muscles and the mitral valve zone of coaptation away from the outflow tract.

Papillary muscle reorientation is most valuable in patients with limited septal hypertrophy, for whom an aggressive myectomy carries increased risk of iatrogenic ventricular septal defect or complete heart block. Anatomically, candidates have hypermobile, bifid papillary muscles that predispose to SAM. Additionally, patients must have a posteriorly positioned papillary muscle, which is fixed to the posterior wall of the ventricle, to allow for relocation and fixation of more anteriorly positioned muscle heads. We have found that fixation of a papillary muscle to the muscle of the posterior left ventricular wall is prone to failure.

MITRAL VALVE REPLACEMENT

Mitral valve replacement has long been known to alleviate LVOT obstruction in HOCM. Excision or posterior translocation of the anterior mitral leaflet eliminates the possibility of SAM and effectively opens the outflow tract [13, 14]. However, with adequate myectomy and the appropriate use of other mitral valve interventions, mitral valve replacement has become the procedure of last resort. In the modern era, mitral valve replacement should be reserved for patients with irreparable intrinsic valve disease or mitral stenosis, prior myectomy, or persistent LVOT obstruction after all other options have been exhausted.

Over 11 years at Cleveland Clinic, only 2.7% of patients required mitral valve replacement of LVOT obstruction [9]. In this series, there was no difference in hemodynamic outcomes between patients receiving mechanical or bioprosthetic valves. If a biologic valve is chosen, care should be taken to ensure that the struts are oriented away from the outflow tract.

REFERENCES

1. Jiang L, Levine RA, King ME, and Weyman AE. An integrated mechanism for systolic anterior motion of the mitral valve in hypertrophic cardiomyopathy based on echocardiographic observations. *Am Heart J.* 1987;113:633.
2. Levine RA, Vlahakes GJ, Lefebvre X, et al. Papillary muscle displacement causes systolic anterior motion of the mitral valve. *Circulation.* 1995;91:1189–1195.
3. Klues HG, Maron BJ, Dollar AL, and Roberts WC. Diversity of structural mitral valve alterations in hypertrophic cardiomyopathy. *Circulation.* 1992;85:1651–1660.
4. Maron MS, Olivotto I, Harrigan C, et al. Mitral valve abnormalities identified by cardiovascular magnetic resonance represents primary phenotypic expression of hypertrophic cardiomyopathy. *Circulation.* 2011;124:40–47.
5. Patel P, Dhillon A, Popovic ZB, et al. Left ventricular outflow tract obstruction in hypertrophic cardiomyopathy patients without severe septal hypertrophy. *Circ Cardiovasc Imaging.* 2015;8:e003132.
6. Wei LM, Thibault DP, Rankin JS, et al. Contemporary surgical management of hypertrophic cardiomyopathy in the United States. *Ann Thorac Surg.* 2019;107:460–466.
7. Hong JH, Schaff HV, Nishimura RA, et al. Mitral regurgitation in patients with hypertrophic obstructive cardiomyopathy. *J Am Coll Cardiol.* 2016;68:1497–1504.
8. Nguyen A, Schaff HV, Nishimura RA, et al. Does septal thickness influence outcome of myectomy for hypertrophic obstructive cardiomyopathy? *Eur J Cardiothorac Surg.* 2018;53:582–589.
9. Hodges K, Godoy Rivas C, Aguilera J, et al. Surgical management of left ventricular outflow tract obstruction in a specialized hypertrophic obstructive cardiomyopathy center. *J Thorac Cardiovasc Surg.* 2019;157:2289–2299.
10. Ferrazzi P, Spirito P, Iacovoni A, et al. Transaortic chordal cutting: Mitral valve repair of obstructive hypertrophic cardiomyopathy with mild septal hypertrophy. *J Am CollCardiol.* 2015;66:1687–1696.

11. Kwon DH, Smedira NG, Thamilarasa M, et al. Characteristics and surgical outcomes of symptomatic patients with hypertrophic cardiomyopathy with abnormal papillary muscle morphology undergoing papillary muscle reorientation. *J Thorac Cardiovasc Surg.* 2010;140:317–324.

12. Song HK, Turner J, Macfie R, et al. Routine papillary muscle realignment and septal myectomy for obstructive hypertrophic cardiomyopathy. *Ann Thorac Surg.* 2018;106:670–675.

13. McIntosh CL, Greenberg GJ, Maron BJ, et al. Clinical and hemodynamic results after mitral valve replacement in patients with obstructive hypertrophic cardiomyopathy. *Ann Thorac Surg.* 1989;47(2):236–246.

14. Leachman RD, Krajcer Z, Azic T, and Cooley DA. Mitral valve replacement in hypertrophic cardiomyopathy: Ten-year follow-up in 54 patients. *Am J Cardiol.* 1987;60:1416–1418.

Chapter 8

ANESTHETIC MANAGEMENT FOR SURGICAL MYECTOMY IN HYPERTROPHIC CARDIOMYOPATHY

Heather K. Hayanga, Jeremiah W. Hayanga, Joseph McGuire, and Vinay Badhwar

CONTENTS

INTRODUCTION

Hypertrophic cardiomyopathy (HCM) is the most common genetic cardiovascular disease transmitted as an autosomal dominant trait [1]. Cardiomyopathy (CM) involves 14 genes with approximately 1,400 mutations that affect sarcomere protein mutations and results in exuberant left ventricular hypertrophy (LVH) [1–6]. Based on mixed epidemiologic studies, the prevalence of phenotypically expressed HCM in the adult general population is estimated at 0.2% (1,500) [1–5]. The majority of afflicted patients live a near-normal life span but are, nevertheless, susceptible to sudden cardiac death, symptoms secondary to dynamic left ventricular outflow tract obstruction (LVOTO), abnormal diastolic filling, impaired left ventricular systolic function, and atrial fibrillation. Each of these may preclude normal physical activities and impair quality and even duration of life [7].

Hypertrophic cardiomyopathy is considered to be non-dilated LVH in the absence of other causes of LVH. Left ventricular wall thickness greater than 15 mm indicates HCM [6]. Subclinical HCM refers to genotype-positive disease without phenotypic expression [8]. Differential diagnoses include aortic stenosis, systemic hypertension, infiltrative diseases, athlete's heart, and metabolic storage disorders (e.g., Fabry's disease or Noonan's syndrome) [6, 9]. Although CMR has great utility in the diagnostic process, echocardiography is still the most commonly used modality [7, 10].

The clinical stages may be classified into four [6]:

- Stage 1 (subclinical HCM): Genotype positive without phenotype expression.
- Stage 2 (classic HCM): Elevated ejection fraction (EF) > 65%, and late gadolinium enhancement (LGE) denoting myocardial fibrosis, accounts for < 5% of left ventricular mass. Note the vast majority of patients will have LVOTO at rest or on provocation.
- Stage 3 (adverse remodeling): EF 50–65%, LGE 10–15%.
- Stage 4 (overt dysfunction or end-stage disease): EF < 50%, LGE > 25%, dilated or restrictive cardiomyopathy, LVOTO may be absent.

Left ventricular outflow tract obstruction and significant mitral regurgitation may not be identifiable without provocation.

Surgery performed for myectomy has evolved since it was first performed in London in 1963 [11]. The technique consisted of an incision into the muscular ridge of the septum [11]. This evolved further and surgical myectomy has now become the gold standard for HCM with LVOTO [12]. There is also growing interest in a minimally invasive approach via the left atrium [13]. The resection involves two longitudinal incisions into the septum, beneath the right coronary cusp as well as beneath the commissure between the left and right coronary cusps. The incisions are connected superiorly with a third incision below the aortic valve that permits the careful resection of a deep wedge of septal tissue extended beyond the point of mitral–septal contact [10].

There are unique challenges in managing these patients under anesthesia and it is necessary and worthwhile for the anesthesiologist to become familiar with the hemodynamic goals and disease-specific nuances associated with the management of these patients in both cardiac and non-cardiac operative settings.

PREOPERATIVE ANESTHETIC EVALUATION

The diagnosis may be made from a combination of history, physical examination, and echocardiographic and/or conventional imaging that highlights the obstructive pathology showing LVH is not attributable to another disease process. In patients who already have a diagnosis of HCM, a standard preoperative history and physical will be necessary. The history should provide answers to the specific questions pertaining to clinical presentation that led to the diagnosis as well as a history of arrhythmias. Symptoms may include impaired exercise capacity, dyspnea on exertion, angina, lightheadedness, or prior syncopal episodes [14]. Medications including chronic beta blockers or calcium channel blockers should be continued [15]. On physical examination, a characteristic harsh crescendo-decrescendo systolic murmur may be auscultated on the left sternal border. This does not radiate to carotids but is accentuated by any decrease in preload [10, 16]. Furthermore, a displaced cardiac apex, and third or fourth heart sounds, may be appreciated [14].

Chest radiography may reveal an enlarged heart. Electrocardiography changes are often nonspecific but may include increased QRS voltage, LVH, and left-axis deviation [10]. Transthoracic echocardiography (TTE) is the primary screening tool and will typically reflect increases in left ventricular wall thickness as well as any alterations in diastolic function [6]. For LVOTO, pulsed-wave Doppler sampling of the left ventricular cavity from the subaortic valve area to the apex may be used to identify the precise location of obstruction, whereas continuous-wave Doppler results will serve to quantify the peak gradient [7, 17]. Interrogation of the mitral valve may identify systolic anterior motion (SAM) of the valve leaflets and chordae, further worsening LVOTO and distorting leaflet coaptation, causing mitral regurgitation. Other imaging modalities may have been completed during the work-up, such as cardiovascular magnetic resonance (CMR), as an alternative in the assessment of cardiac structure, function, and severity of LVOTO. These should also be carefully reviewed.

CARDIOVASCULAR IMPLANTABLE ELECTRONIC DEVICES

Patients with HCM often present preoperatively with an automated implantable cardioverter defibrillator (AICD) in view of the concomitant propensity for ventricular arrhythmias and sudden cardiac death [2]. Once it is determined that the patient has an AICD, electrophysiology services should be sought to discontinue anti-tachyarrhythmia therapies intraoperatively. Preoperative electrocardiography should be reviewed to determine if the patient is also dependent on the pacemaker component of the AICD, and if so, the AICD should be placed in an asynchronous mode for the duration of the operation given the high likelihood of electromagnetic interference. External defibrillator pads should be placed and remain *in situ* until the AICD is reprogrammed postoperatively. Any pre-inserted DDD pacemaker placed for timed atrial contraction and gradient reduction should not be inactivated [18].

INTRAOPERATIVE CONSIDERATIONS

INDUCTION OF ANESTHESIA

Induction of anesthesia must cater to the hemodynamic goals of HCM, namely avoiding aggravation of LVOTO and remaining cognizant of diastolic dysfunction that may be less amenable to direct pharmacologic manipulation [15]. Hypertrophic cardiomyopathy with LVOTO is a dynamic process, one that is altered by changes in preload, afterload, heart rate, and cardiac contractility. A pre-induction arterial line should be placed, and standard monitoring should be used. Given that the patient has likely been *nil per os*, standardly for the preceding eight hours or perhaps two hours depending on the use of enhanced recovery after cardiac surgery (ERACS) protocols, he or she is likely to be volume depleted prior to surgery. Taking into consideration the patient's left ventricular function, a modest bolus of crystalloid prior to induction may be used to optimize preload prior to administering anesthetic medications. Regardless of the induction medication used, maintaining afterload will be imperative to ensure appropriate coronary perfusion pressure to the hypertrophied left ventricle. Heart rate should be kept low and rhythm normal to allow for adequate diastolic filling to then maximize ejection with minimal turbulence in the left ventricular outflow tract (LVOT). Attempt to minimize preoperative anxiety. A deep level of general anesthesia will minimize tachycardia as well as increases in contractility associated with intubation and surgical stimulation [15]. Cardiac contractility should be maintained with an aim towards mild myocardial depression as an increase in contractility will lead to increased dynamic outflow tract obstruction, thereby limiting ejection. Indeed, low dose beta-blockade may be used to mitigate tachycardia during laryngoscopy and are additionally beneficial for their negative inotropic effect [10] (Figure 8.1).

MAINTENANCE OF ANESTHESIA

Anticipated sympathetic stimulation from the surgery should be minimized using multimodal analgesia and inhalation anesthetics. Sevoflurane, as opposed to isoflurane or desflurane, is best suited for maintenance of anesthesia due to its minimal effect on heart rate and systemic vascular resistance (SVR) [9]. The inhalation anesthetics are commonly used in HCM, given their dose-dependent myocardial depression [15]. Nitrous oxide enhances sympathetic stimulation and potentially elevates pulmonary vascular resistance. As such, it should be avoided [10]. Dexmedotomidine reduces heart rate and blocks sympathetic stimulation but may result in hypotension, and thus must be used judiciously [10]. Non-depolarizing neuromuscular blocking agents that do not cause histamine release, such as vecuronium or rocuronium, should be used to avoid hypotension and tachycardia.

Low tidal volume ventilation and modest levels of positive end expiratory pressure (PEEP) are recommended and help mitigate the effects of LVOTO [10]. Central venous pressure will likely not reflect accurate left-sided filling pressures due to diastolic dysfunction [10]. Supraventricular or junctional tachyarrhthmias with associated hypotension will require immediate synchronized cardioversion [15]. Synchronized cardioversion should be used to treat any ensuing atrial fibrillation as amiodarone and other pharmacologic agents are slower in action and can result in hypotension [10].

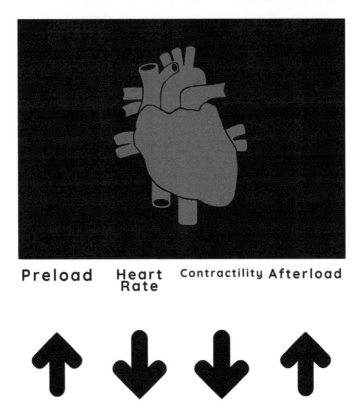

Figure 8.1   Anesthetic management goals for HCM.

Hypotension is often the result of underlying hypovolemia, potentially exacerbated by anesthetic-induced vasodilation [15]. In addition to maintaining an adequate intravascular volume, vasoconstrictors, specifically alpha-adrenergic agonists such as phenylephrine, should preferentially be used rather than inotropes, given its ability to increase systemic vascular resistance with concomitant reflexive bradycardia [1, 10, 19]. Epinephrine is particularly deleterious due to its exacerbation of LVOTO and its positive chronotropic effect [20]. This is true also for anticholinergics that may stimulate tachycardia [1, 10].

INTRAOPERATIVE TRANSESOPHAGEAL ECHOCARDIOGRAPHY

Transesophageal echocardiography (TEE) performed prior to cardiopulmonary bypass should reconfirm preoperative echocardiographic findings and help guide the surgical plan. A comprehensive TEE evaluation should be performed. Asymmetric septal hypertrophy is a consistent finding, but concentric hypertrophy or hypertrophy isolated to other segmental distributions may also be seen [7].

Left ventricular wall thickness typically exceeds 15 mm in HCM, though this may even exceed 20 mm. A thickness greater than 30 mm is considered "massive hypertrophy" [6]. The ventricular thickening is asymmetric and may involve the free wall, apex, and anterolateral wall, and only very rarely is there uniform or concentric hypertrophy of the basal and mid-anterior wall [6]. A few common patterns of HCM have been identified: reverse curvature septum, sigmoid septum, neutral septum, apical septum, and mid-ventricular HCM [6]. These patterns are best viewed in the mid-esophageal (ME) five-chamber view or ME long-axis views. The LVH and the wall thickness may also be assessed in the transgastric (TG) short-axis views at the basal, mid-, and apical levels to best delineate the pattern of hypertrophy. The hypertrophied ventricular walls may obliterate the left ventricular cavity during systole [21]. In the transgastric mid-papillary view, inferolateral wall thickness may be evaluated. A ratio of the septal wall to the inferolateral wall thickness of > 1.3 is reflective of asymmetric septal hypertrophy in non-hypertensive patients. In the case of hypertensive patients, the ratio must exceed 1.5 to qualify as asymmetric hypertrophy [6, 22].

For dynamic obstruction, color-flow Doppler will display turbulence in the LVOT. A late-peaking, dagger-shaped waveform will be appreciated using continuous-wave Doppler through the aortic valve, in either the deep transgastric or transgastric long-axis view(s) [9, 10, 15]. Asymmetric hypertrophy, a prominent basal septum, narrowing of the ventricular cavity, and mitral valve apparatus structural abnormalities all increase the likelihood of LVOTO in HCM [14]. Using M-mode in the ME long-axis view, LVOTO can be observed as the valve leaflets open normally, close prematurely in mid-systole, and then reopen as final ejection occurs [14] (Figure 8.2). Intraoperative measurement of left ventricular end-diastolic pressure and intra-aortic pressure may provide useful additional intraoperative data that may guide the surgeon in estimating the magnitude of myectomy necessary [23].

Diastolic dysfunction occurs in almost all patients with HCM [14, 15]. Reduced systolic and diastolic velocities may be assessed using tissue Doppler imaging (TDI) [7]. Reduction in systolic velocity in the presence of a normal or elevated ejection fraction is highly suggestive of HCM. Mitral annular systolic velocity < 4 m/s serves as an independent predictor of heart failure and mortality [7, 21, 22, 24–26]. Notably, in aortic stenosis, acceleration decreases as velocity increases. In obstructive HCM, however, as velocity increases so too does acceleration [10].

Structural anomalies of the mitral valve in HCM may exacerbate the overlap of the inflow and outflow portions of the left ventricle. This results in coaptation of the body of the leaflets rather than the tips. The anterior mitral leaflet (AML) most commonly makes contact with the septum. The longer the contact between the valve and the septum, the higher the gradient. The ME long-axis view or the ME five-chamber view may be used to measure leaflet lengths. The most

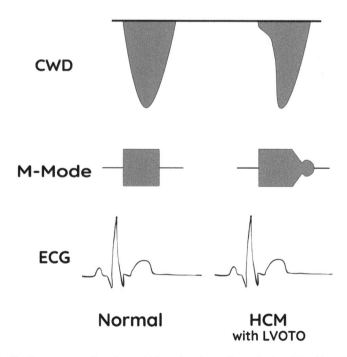

Figure 8.2 Continuous-wave Doppler and M-mode echocardiography in HCM with LVOTO.

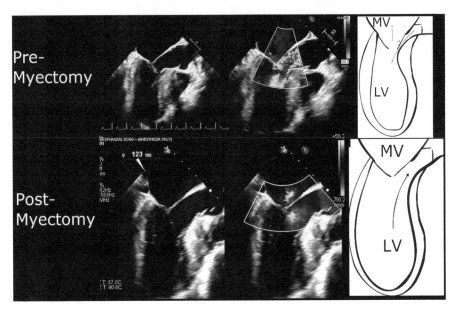

Figure 8.3 Mid-esophageal long-axis transesophageal echocardiography view with and without color-flow Doppler pre- and post-myectomy in patient with SAM of the mitral valve with LVOTO in the setting of HCM.

reproducible way to measure the AML is to do so by measuring the length from its tip to the point of insertion of the non-coronary cusp of the aortic valve [13]. Patients with AML length > 33 mm are candidates for horizontal AML plication. Leaflet calcification, however, represents a contraindication to this type of repair. Patients with AML length > 40 mm may benefit from the resection of the terminal portion of the AML or an Alfieri repair [10, 27, 28]. The coaptation zone between the two leaflets is best seen using the deep transgastric view [10].

Systolic anterior motion of the mitral valve exacerbates the coaptation gap between the leaflets. This is predominately due the discrepancy in the ability of the posterior mitral leaflet (PML) to move towards the outflow tract in comparison to the AML. The mitral regurgitation jet is directed laterally and posteriorly during mid- and late systole. This is typical in obstructive HCM. The MR is thus typically a secondary phenomenon. Risk factors for SAM include redundant or elongated mitral valve leaflets (AML > 2 cm or anterior: posterior leaflet heights from annulus to coaptation point are ≤ 1.3 cm), anteriorly positioned papillary muscles, and a distance between the mitral valve coaptation point and ventricular septum (C-sept distance) of less than 2.5 cm [14] (Figure 8.3). When, however, the MR jet is directed anteriorly, then other causes of MR should be considered, such as mitral valve prolapse, chordal elongation, chordal thickening, or infective endocarditis [7, 10, 29]. Concomitant MV surgery is rarely required but, when necessary, repair is preferred over replacement due to better than ten-year survival (80 vs. 55.2%) [30].

POST-CARDIOPULMONARY BYPASS CONSIDERATIONS

Transesophageal echocardiography allows evaluation of the adequacy of myectomy and any post-operative complications immediately following cardiopulmonary bypass. The LVOT postoperatively should appear widened with improvements in SAM of the mitral valve, MR, and LVOT gradient. Color-flow Doppler should show laminar systolic LVOT flow. Where there is a persistent elevated outflow gradient, one should look for persistent mitral valve or papillary muscle abnormalities. Mitral or aortic regurgitant jets should be measured and evaluated for size, duration, location, and mechanism. The zone of coaptation is best evaluated in the deep transgastric view. A coaptation zone of greater than 5 mm is required for adequate valve closure [8]. Postoperative complications associated with surgical myectomy include atrial arrhythmias, ventricular arrhythmias, heart block, left ventricular rupture, and ventricular septal defect [9]. Excessive resection of the septum may result in a ventricular septal defect (VSD) and this is a consideration that must be borne in mind for a few days postoperatively. As such the septum should be carefully evaluated in the ME views. Flow across the interventricular septum should be differentiated from flow related to unroofed septal perforators, the latter of which will be seen only in diastole. A small amount of residual SAM is permissible and typically resolves within two weeks [28, 31–37].

HYPERTROPHIC CARDIOMYOPATHY IN NON-CARDIAC SURGERY

All the considerations above apply to non-cardiac surgery. However, the use of pneumoperitoneum in laparoscopic surgery and management of the parturient require special mention. The effect of hypercapnia and elevated intra-abdominal pressure may reduce venous return and decrease preload with pneumoperitoneum in laparoscopic surgery. As such, intra-abdominal pressure should be carefully monitored to maintain values less than 15 mm Hg [38]. The hemodynamic changes of pregnancy result in decreased SVR, increase in blood volume, and compression of the aorta and inferior vena cava, particularly in the last trimester. Major blood loss during labor may further exacerbate LVOTO. Oxytocin reduces SVR and increases the heart rate. Careful fluid resuscitation is necessary to optimize anesthetic management of a parturient with HCM, but to also avoid subsequent pulmonary edema with autotransfusion of uterine blood, leading to increased peripheral vascular resistance in the immediate post-delivery period. Although neuraxial anesthesia may reduce preload and afterload from vasodilation and sympathetic blockade, intrathecal and epidural anesthesia in pregnant patients with HCM have been safely provided [10, 38].

CONCLUSION

Hypertrophic cardiomyopathy is a common genetic cardiovascular disorder. Surgical repair poses unique challenges for the cardiac anesthesiologist but with careful and thoughtful consideration of the prevailing physiologic milieu, a safe and reproducible algorithm of care may be achieved utilizing TEE and select pharmacologic agents to ensure safe outcomes.

REFERENCES

1. Poliac LC, Barron ME, Maron BJ. Hypertrophic cardiomyopathy. *Anesthesiology* 2006. https://doi.org/10.1097/00000542-200601000-00025.
2. Trivedi A, Knight BP. ICD therapy for primary prevention in hypertrophic cardiomyopathy. *Arrhythmia Electrophysiol Rev* 2016. https://doi.org/10.15420/aer.2016:30:2.
3. Maron BJ, Ommen SR, Semsarian C, Spirito P, Olivotto I, Maron MS. Hypertrophic cardiomyopathy: Present and future, with translation into contemporary cardiovascular medicine. *J Am Coll Cardiol* 2014. https://doi.org/10.1016/j.jacc.2014.05.003.
4. Maron BJ, Gardin JM, Flack JM, Gidding SS, Kurosaki TT, Bild DE. Prevalence of hypertrophic cardiomyopathy in a general population of young adults: Echocardiographic analysis of 4111 subjects in the CARDIA study. *Circulation* 1995. https://doi.org/10.1161/01.CIR.92.4.785.
5. Wheeler M, Pavlovic A, Degoma E, Salisbury H, Brown C, Ashley EA. A new era in clinical genetic testing for hypertrophic cardiomyopathy. *J Cardiovasc Transl Res* 2009. https://doi.org/10.1007/s12265-009-9139-0.
6. Varma P, Neema P. Hypertrophic cardiomyopathy: Part 1–Introduction, pathology and pathophysiology. *Ann Card Anaesth* 2014. https://doi.org/10.4103/0971-9784.129841.

7. Nagueh SF, Bierig SM, Budoff MJ, Desai M, Dilsizian V, Eidem B, et al. American society of echocardiography clinical recommendations for multimodality cardiovascular imaging of patients with hypertrophic cardiomyopathy: Endorsed by the American Society of Nuclear Cardiology, Society for Cardiovascular Magnetic Resonance, and Society of Cardiovascular Computed Tomography. *J Am Soc Echocardiogr* 2011. https://doi.org/10.1016/j.echo.2011.03.006.

8. Gersh BJ, Maron BJ, Bonow RO, Dearani JA, Fifer MA, Link MS, et al. 2011 ACCF/AHA guideline for the diagnosis and treatment of hypertrophic cardiomyopathy: A report of the American College of Cardiology Foundation/American Heart Association Task Force on practice guidelines. *Circulation* 2011. https://doi.org/10.1161/CIR.0b013e318223e2bd.

9. Vegas A. *Perioperative two-dimensional transesophageal echocardiography: A practical handbook.* 2nd ed., Springer; 2018, pp. 310–313.

10. Varma PK, Raman SP, Neema PK. Hypertrophic cardiomyopathy part II - Anesthetic and surgical considerations. *Ann Card Anaesth* 2014. https://doi.org/10.4103/0971-9784.135852.

11. Cleland WP. The surgical management of obstructive cardiomyopathy. *J Cardiovasc Surg (Torino)* 1963.

12. Morrow AG, Reitz BA, Epstein SE, Henry WL, Conkle DM, Itscoitz SB, et al. Operative treatment in hypertrophic subaortic stenosis. Techniques, and the results of pre and postoperative assessments in 83 patients. *Circulation* 1975. https://doi.org/10.1161/01.CIR.52.1.88.

13. Mohr FW, Seeburger J, Misfeld M. Keynote Lecture-Transmitral hypertrophic obstructive cardiomyopathy (HOCM) repair. *Ann Cardiothorac Surg* 2013. https://doi.org/10.3978/j.issn.2225-319X.2013.11.05.

14. Prabhu M, Roysam C, Shernan S. Ventricular diseases. In: Mathew J, Ayoub C, Nicoara A, Swaminathan M, editors. *Clin Man Rev Transesophageal Echocardiogram.* 3rd ed., McGraw Hill Education; 2019, pp. 548–577.

15. Ramakrishna H, Craner R, Devaleria P, Cook D, Housmans P, Rehfeldt K. Valvular heart disease: Replacement and repair. In: Kaplan J, Cronin B, Maus T, editors. *Card Surg Essentials Card Anesth*, Elsevier; 2018, pp. 352–384.

16. Malani PN. Harrison's Principles of Internal Medicine. *JAMA* 2012. https://doi.org/10.1001/jama.308.17.1813-b.

17. Sleilaty G, El-Rassi I, Jebara V, Swaminathan M. *Clinical Manual and Review of Transesophageal Echocardiography.* 3rd ed., McGraw Hill Education; 2019.

18. Jain A, Jain K, Bhagat H, Mangal K, Batra Y. Anesthetic management of a patient with hypertrophic obstructive cardiomyopathy with dual-chamber pacemaker undergoing transurethral resection of the prostate. *Ann Card Anaesth* 2010. https://doi.org/10.4103/0971-9784.69043.

19. Gajewski M, Hillel Z. Anesthesia management of patients with hypertrophic obstructive cardiomyopathy. *Prog Cardiovasc Dis* 2012. https://doi.org/10.1016/j.pcad.2012.04.002.

20. Yee KFH, Wąsowicz M. Anaphylaxis and cardiac surgery for hypertrophic obstructive cardiomyopathy: A case report and review of anaesthetic management. *Anaesthesiol Intensive Ther* 2016. https://doi.org/10.5603/AIT.a2016.0042.

21. Lang RM, Bierig M, Devereux RB, Flachskampf FA, Foster E, Pellikka PA, et al. Recommendations for chamber quantification: A report from the American Society of Echocardiography's guidelines and standards committee and the Chamber Quantification Writing Group, developed in conjunction with the European Association of Echocardiograph. *J Am Soc Echocardiogr* 2005. https://doi.org/10.1016/j.echo.2005.10.005.

22. Williams LK, Frenneaux MP, Steeds RP. Echocardiography in hypertrophic cardiomyopathy diagnosis, prognosis, and role in management. *Eur J Echocardiogr* 2009. https://doi.org/10.1093/ejechocard/jep157.

23. Ashikhmina EA, Schaff HV, Ommen SR, Dearani JA, Nishimura RA, Abel MD. Intraoperative direct measurement of left ventricular outflow tract gradients to guide surgical myectomy for hypertrophic cardiomyopathy. *J Thorac Cardiovasc Surg* 2011. https://doi.org/10.1016/j.jtcvs.2010.08.011.

24. Cardim N, Perrot A, Ferreira T, Pereira A, Osterziel KJ, Palma Reis R, et al. Usefulness of Doppler myocardial imaging for identification of mutation carriers of familial hypertrophic cardiomyopathy. *Am J Cardiol* 2002. https://doi.org/10.1016/S0002-9149(02)02434-7.

25. Bayrak F, Kahveci G, Mutlu B, Sonmez K, Degertekin M. Tissue Doppler imaging to predict clinical course of patients with hypertrophic cardiomyopathy. *Eur J Echocardiogr* 2008. https://doi.org/10.1093/ejechocard/jen049.

26. Kato TS, Noda A, Izawa H, Yamada A, Obata K, Nagata K, et al. Discrimination of non-obstructive hypertrophic cardiomyopathy from hypertensive left ventricular hypertrophy on the basis of strain rate imaging by tissue Doppler ultrasonography. *Circulation* 2004. https://doi.org/10.1161/01.CIR.0000150334.69355.00.

27. Sherrid MV, Arabadjian M. Echocardiography to individualize treatment for hypertrophic cardiomyopathy. *Prog Cardiovasc Dis* 2012. https://doi.org/10.1016/j.pcad.2012.04.007.

28. Swistel DG, Balaram SK. Surgical myectomy for hypertrophic cardiomyopathy in the 21st century, the evolution of the "RPR" repair: Resection, plication, and release. *Prog Cardiovasc Dis* 2012. https://doi.org/10.1016/j.pcad.2012.03.001.

29. DiNardo JA, Zvara DA. *Anesthesia for Cardiac Surgery*. 3rd ed. Massachusetts: Blackwell Publishing; 2008.

30. Hong JH, Schaff HV, Nishimura RA, Abel MD, Dearani JA, Li Z, et al. Mitral regurgitation in patients with hypertrophic obstructive cardiomyopathy: Implications for concomitant valve procedures. *J Am Coll Cardiol* 2016. https://doi.org/10.1016/j.jacc.2016.07.735.

31. Nakamura T, Matsubara K, Furukawa K, Azuma A, Sugihara H, Katsume H, et al. Diastolic paradoxic jet flow in patients with hypertrophic cardiomyopathy: Evidence of concealed apical asynergy with cavity obliteration. *J Am Coll Cardiol* 1992. https://doi.org/10.1016/S0735-1097(10)80264-5.

32. Fischer GW, Anyanwu AC, Adams DH. Intraoperative classification of mitral valve dysfunction: The role of the anesthesiologist in mitral valve reconstruction. *J Cardiothorac Vasc Anesth* 2009. https://doi.org/10.1053/j.jvca.2009.03.002.

33. Bartels K, Daneshmand MA, Mathew JP, Glower DD, Swaminathan M, Nicoara A. Delayed postmyectomy ventricular septal defect. *J Cardiothorac Vasc Anesth* 2013. https://doi.org/10.1053/j.jvca.2012.10.009.

34. Siegman IL, Maron BJ, Permut LC, McIntosh CL, Clark RE. Results of operation for coexistent obstructive hypertrophic cardiomyopathy and coronary artery disease. *J Am Coll Cardiol* 1989. https://doi.org/10.1016/0735-1097(89)90343-4.

35. Dhillon A, Khanna A, Randhawa MS, Cywinski J, Saager L, Thamilarasan M, et al. Perioperative outcomes of patients with hypertrophic cardiomyopathy undergoing non-cardiac surgery. *Heart* 2016. https://doi.org/10.1136/heartjnl-2016-309442.

36. Swaminathan S, Qirko K, Smith T, Corcoran E, Wysham NG, Bazaz G, et al. A machine learning approach to triaging patients with chronic obstructive pulmonary disease. *PLoS One* 2017. https://doi.org/10.1371/journal.pone.0188532.

37. Ommen SR, Park SH, Click RL, Freeman WK, Schaff H V., Tajik AJ. Impact of intraoperative transesophageal echocardiography in the surgical management of hypertrophic cardiomyopathy. *Am J Cardiol* 2002. https://doi.org/10.1016/S0002-9149(02)02694-2.

38. Ishiyama T, Oguchi T, Iijima T, Matsukawa T, Kashimoto S, Kumazawa T. Combined spinal and epidural anesthesia for cesarean section in a patient with hypertrophic obstructive cardiomyopathy. *Anesth Analg* 2003. https://doi.org/10.1213/00000539-200302000-00067.

Chapter 9

COMPLICATIONS OF SEPTAL MYECTOMY

Lawrence M. Wei, Charlotte Spear, and Vinay Badhwar

CONTENTS

INTRODUCTION

Septal myectomy is the primary surgical therapy for the management of hypertrophic cardiomyopathy (HCM) with obstruction. Following Brock's description in 1957 of the obstructive nature of HCM [1], surgeons soon recognized that the underlying anatomical abnormality favored a surgical solution. By 1961, Kirklin and Ellis [2], as well as Morrow and Brockenbrough [3], had established the technique of subaortic resection of the muscular ventricular septum and described the original technique of removing a narrow bar of septal myocardium. The operation has since been refined methodically to include a wider and more apically directed resection and now commonly is described as *extended septal myectomy* (Figure 9.1).

Extended septal myectomy effectively relieves symptoms of heart failure by eliminating left ventricular outflow tract (LVOT) obstruction and mitral valve (MV) regurgitation. The operation improves functional capacity, quality of life, and survival [4, 5]. Patients undergoing septal myectomy have a long-term survival that is comparable to the general population [5]. Surgical septal myectomy is widely recognized as the gold standard of treatment of HCM inpatients with obstructive symptoms refractory to medical therapy who are able to undergo surgery.

Septal myectomy is a safe and reproducible operation in the hands of experienced operators. Most operations for HCM in the United States are performed at a small number of institutions [6]. Experienced institutions have reported good short-term outcomes and low operative mortality, in some instances less than 0.5% [7–9]. A study of surgical management of HCM in the United States based on data from the Society of Thoracic Surgeons Adult Cardiac Surgery Database showed that operative mortality for septal myectomy without concomitant MV operation was 1.6% [6], though another study deriving information from the National Inpatient Sample showed an overall mortality of 5.9% [10] for all septal myectomy procedures.

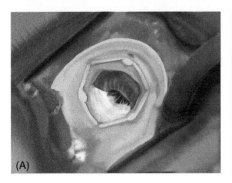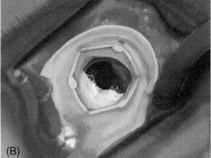

(A)　　　　　　　　　　　　　　(B)

Figure 9.1　Surgeon's view of left ventricular outflow tract. (A) Before myectomy. (B) After extended septal myectomy.

COMPLICATIONS

Complications of the surgical treatment of HCM may include those associated with the conduct of any cardiac operation, as well as those specific to septal myectomy. Avoidance of complications specific to septal myectomy is dependent on a detailed understanding of the anatomy and pathophysiology of HCM and the technical details of the operation.

The subaortic LVOT is bounded anteriorly by the ventricular septum and posteriorly by the anterior leaflet of the MV. The aortic valve defines the exit of the LVOT and a significant portion of the conduction system lies within the septum (Figure 9.2). These structures bounding the LVOT are potentially at risk for injury during septal myectomy and most complications are related to incidental injury to the anatomy.

RHYTHM ABNORMALITIES

Patients with HCM undergoing septal myectomy may have pre-existing underlying conduction abnormalities that may predispose them to complete heart block. Septal myectomy, correctly performed, resects myocardium that may include the left bundle of His, and a left bundle branch block pattern commonly is present on a postoperative electrocardiogram. If the right bundle branch block is present before surgery, as is common in HCM patients with prior alcohol septal ablation, complete heart block (CHB) may be unavoidable.

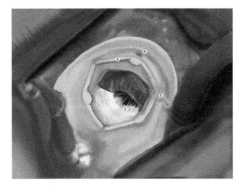

Figure 9.2　Structures adjacent to LVOT. (1) Conduction system. (2) Anterior leaflet of mitral valve. (3) Right coronary cusp of aortic valve. (4) Right coronary ostium.

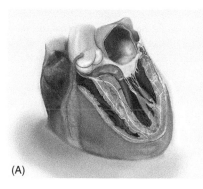 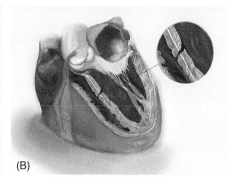

(A)   (B)

Figure 9.3 Ventricular septal defect. (A) Correct depth of resection for septal myectomy. (B) Ventricular septal defect from excessively deep resection.

Complete heart block requiring implantation of a permanent pacemaker is a well-known complication of septal myectomy. The incidence of postoperative pacemaker implantation has been reported as less than 5% in large series of septal myectomy [6, 7, 11]. This compares favorably with alcohol septal ablation, which carries a risk of 10–15% for heart block, requiring implantation of a permanent pacemaker [12], which has significant consequences for the patient undergoing cardiac surgery. The need for a permanent pacemaker after surgical aortic valve replacement (AVR) may reduce long-term survival [13]. Permanent pacemaker implantation in patients undergoing septal myectomy, who are younger on average than those undergoing AVR, may be subject to secondary long-term deleterious effects.

Patients with normal atrioventricular (AV) conduction before surgery should not develop CHB from septal myectomy. Injury to the AV node and resultant CHB may be avoided by careful attention to the limits of muscular resection. The medial extent of the sub-annular portion of the resection should be limited to the nadir of the right coronary sinus, below the ostium of the right coronary artery. If additional medial resection of the septum is necessary, it should be performed more apically, at a safe distance from the membranous septum and AV node (Figure 9.3(A)). Patients undergoing septal myectomy should have temporary epicardial pacemaker leads placed during surgery. If the AV block persists in the postoperative period, a permanent dual-chamber pacemaker should be implanted prior to discharge.

A patient with an extremely thick septum or high degree of LVOT obstruction may be at elevated risk of ventricular arrhythmias and sudden cardiac death (SCD). Septal myectomy (SM) may actually reduce the risk of ventricular arrhythmia [14]. If the risk of such arrhythmia and SCD is judged to be high, an implantable cardioverter-defibrillator (ICD) should be placed. Alternatively, the patient at risk may be discharged with a wearable external defibrillator.

Atrial fibrillation (AF) occurs commonly in the postoperative period of septal myectomy as it does for all other cardiac operations. Even after a successful septal myectomy with full relief of LVOT obstruction, AF may be poorly tolerated because of diastolic dysfunction and impaired ventricular filling. Aggressive management of postoperative AF including pharmacological therapy and electrical cardioversion is recommended. If AF is present prior to surgery, a concomitant full bi-atrial Cox Maze IV operation should be strongly considered as an adjunct to the septal myectomy.

VENTRICULAR SEPTAL DEFECT

The incidence of iatrogenic ventricular septal defect (VSD) during septal myectomy is less than 1%. If a VSD is recognized during performance of septal myectomy, it should be repaired immediately. Rarely, a new VSD may be noted on late follow-up. If there is significant flow through the defect, it should be repaired. Catheter-based approaches can be useful and may reduce the need for reoperation.

The best approach to managing the complication of a VSD is to not create one. Careful attention to technical precision, including the depth of resection, is the key to preventing this dangerous and potentially fatal complication. With the excellent quality of current cardiac imaging modalities, including transesophageal echocardiography (TEE), computed tomography (CT), and magnetic resonance imaging, precise preoperative mapping of the septal thickness is feasible. This information allows the surgeon to plan and execute the myocardial resection to the correct depth in the septum. Taking the planning a step further, three-dimensional printing of a replica of the patient's heart generated from the CT scan may allow practicing the resection before the actual operation.

A small iatrogenic VSD may be primarily closed, but many VSDs will require a patch of autologous pericardium for repair (Figure 9.3(B)). A VSD discovered postoperatively that is not causing hemodynamic compromise may be left untreated while the tissues heal. The defect may be closed later with an occlusion device delivered via a transcatheter approach once a firm rim of tissue has formed to securely anchor the device.

AORTIC VALVE

Unplanned aortic valve replacement is a rare complication of septal myectomy, occurring in less than 1% of cases. The standard approach to the LVOT septum through the aortic valve creates a risk of injury to the valve. A common technique employed for septal exposure is retraction of the right coronary cusp with a ribbon-shaped retractor. Excessive traction may cause tears in the cusp. The assistant holding the retractor must be careful to retract gently in order to avoid valvular injury. Alternative methods of retracting the valve to expose the septum include using a self-retaining retractor mounted to a flexible mechanical arm or placing a fine monofilament suture through the Nodule of Arantius of the right coronary cusp and temporarily tacking it to the aorta. Regardless of the method used to expose the septum, care must be taken to avoid excessive retraction. An injured valve cusp should be repaired primarily or with autologous pericardium. If repair is not possible, aortic valve replacement must be performed.

Aortic insufficiency may be created inadvertently by unhinging the right coronary cusp. Unhinging occurs when the margin of resection strays too close to the aortic annulus, leaving the right coronary cusp with inadequate support. Prolapse of the cusp occurs and produces aortic insufficiency. This complication can be eliminated by beginning the resection no closer than 5 mm to the aortic annulus. Aortic insufficiency caused by this mechanism may occur late after surgery. An insufficiently unhinged valve may be repaired with a sub-annular annuloplasty ring or may require replacement.

MITRAL VALVE

The mitral valve plays a significant role in the pathophysiology of HCM in many patients. Systolic anterior motion (SAM) of the mitral valve is an important mechanism for creating LVOT obstruction and symptoms of heart failure. The majority of patients with HCM and obstruction have significant MV regurgitation from SAM or, less commonly, due to intrinsic MV pathology [8]. Moreover, injury to the MV apparatus may occur during septal resection. Despite the high incidence of preoperative MV regurgitation in HCM with obstruction, most patients undergoing septal myectomy do not require an MV procedure. Septal myectomy alone eliminates significant MV regurgitation in 85.5% patients [6], and some centers have reported that patients undergoing septal myectomy alone have severe MV regurgitation reduced from a preoperative incidence of 54.3% to 1.7% postoperatively [8].

In the majority of cases, performing an adequate septal myectomy requires extending the resection apically at least to the mid-papillary muscle level. The chordae tendineae of the mitral valve are at risk of injury because of limited visibility deep in the ventricle. The surgeon must be careful to visualize and avoid injuring the chordae during septal resection. Use of a malleable "ribbon" retractor to retract the mitral structures in a posterior direction can be helpful. If a primary chord is injured, MV regurgitation may ensue. The damage may be repaired by transferring a secondary chord, implanting an artificial chord, or performing edge-to-edge leaflet repair. Absent surgical injury, residual MV regurgitation following discontinuation of cardiopulmonary bypass most commonly occurs because insufficient left ventricular muscle has been resected from the septum. Resuming cardiopulmonary bypass and completing the resection will resolve the problem in the vast majority of cases. If significant persistent MV regurgitation remains following re-resection, the valve must be repaired or replaced. Mortality for MV repair is significantly lower than for MV replacement when performed in conjunction with septal myectomy [6, 8]. Standard techniques of MV repair that involve posterior leaflet height reduction are applicable, but unusual mitral pathology including abnormal papillary muscles may be present and must be addressed.

RESIDUAL OBSTRUCTION
Inadequate septal resection can leave a patient not only with residual MV regurgitation, but with residual LVOT obstruction. Following septal myectomy, the surgical result must be assessed to ensure that adequate resection has been achieved. Visualizing and quantifying the elimination of SAM-related MV regurgitation and quantifying the LVOT gradient by TEE is essential to the conduct of the operation. Direct measurement of simultaneous LV and aortic pressures provides an accurate assessment of the LVOT gradient. Employing provocative measures such as administration of inotropic and chronotropic agents ensures that the gradient is measured under the physiologic conditions most likely to produce obstructive LVOT obstruction. If a residual gradient remains after septal myectomy, it must be addressed immediately by performing additional resection. The TEE may be useful in guiding the surgeon to areas requiring additional resection. Often, more apically directed resection is required.

STROKE
Stroke is an inherent risk of all cardiac operations, including septal myectomy. By its nature, septal myectomy creates a large area of raw myocardium with the potential for embolization of myocardial fragments. Resection should leave as smooth a surface on the septum as possible and irregular, shaggy areas must be meticulously debrided. Copious irrigation of the ventricular cavity and evacuation of the irrigation fluid is standard technique. Antiplatelet agents should be administered postoperatively, but long-term oral anticoagulation is not necessary for isolated septal myectomy.

HEMODYNAMIC COMPLICATIONS
Postoperative hemodynamic complications can ensue from improper management of the hypertrophic left ventricle during and after the operation. Protection of the hypertrophic ventricle during the ischemic period is critical. Antegrade cardioplegia provides optimal protection of the myocardium, particularly the subendocardial region, and should be employed either exclusively or in conjunction with retrograde delivery. For an isolated myectomy in the setting of a competent aortic valve, a single dose of antegrade cardioplegia may be sufficient. For more complex procedures, additional doses are needed and may be delivered directly into the coronary ostia. Optimal myocardial protection preserves postoperative biventricular function.

The approach to weaning from cardiopulmonary bypass (CPB) should take into account the pathophysiology of HCM and ensure optimization of coronary perfusion pressure (CPP), which is determined by the difference of the mean arterial pressure (MAP) and the left ventricular end-diastolic pressure (LVEDP) by the equation $CPP = MAP - LVEDP$. Mean arterial pressure should be maintained with volume infusion to ensure adequate preload of the stiff, hypertrophic ventricle and with vasopressor agents, not inotropes, to avoid increasing contractility. This approach will minimize the risk of creating a transient increase in the contractile state that could induce SAM and LVOT obstruction. Maintaining coronary perfusion pressure also is a key to avoiding post-bypass right-ventricular dysfunction.

SUMMARY

Septal myectomy is a safe and reproducible operation that provides excellent outcomes. It is considered to be the gold standard of treatment for patients with HCM and obstructive symptoms refractory to medical therapy. Thorough understanding of the pathoanatomy and pathophysiology of HCM is necessary to achieve successful relief of outflow obstruction. Most complications of septal myectomy can be readily avoided and successful outcomes realized by precise attention to the technical details of the operation and careful hemodynamic management during and after operation.

REFERENCES

1. Brock R. Functional obstruction of the left ventricle. *Guys Hospital Report*, 1957. 106: p. 221–239.
2. Kirklin JW, Ellis FH. Surgical relief of diffuse subvalvular aortic stenosis. *Circulation*, 1961. 24: p. 739–742.
3. Morrow AG, Brockenbrough EC. Surgical treatment of idiopathic hypertrophic subaortic stenosis: Technic and hemodynamic results of subaortic ventriculomyotomy. *Ann Surg*, 1961. 154: p. 181–189.
4. Deb SJ, Schaff HV, Dearani JA, et al. Septal myectomy results in regression of left ventricular hypertrophy in patients with hypertrophic obstructive cardiomyopathy. *Ann Thorac Surg*, 2004. 78(6): p. 2118–2122.
5. Ommen SR, Maron BJ, Olivotto I, et al. Long-term effects of surgical septal myectomy on survival in patients with obstructive hypertrophic cardiomyopathy. *J Am Coll Cardiol*, 2005. 46: p. 470–476.
6. Wei LM, Thibault DP, Rankin JS, et al. Contemporary surgical management of hypertrophic cardiomyopathy in the United States. *Ann Thorac Surg*, 2019. 107(2): p. 460–466.
7. Smedira NG, Lytle BW, Lever HM, et al. Current effectiveness and risks of isolated septal myectomy for hypertrophic obstructive cardiomyopathy. *Ann Thorac Surg*, 2008. 85(1): p. 127–133.
8. Hong JH, Schaff HV, Nishimura RA, et al. Mitral regurgitation in patients with hypertrophic obstructive cardiomyopathy: Implications for concomitant valve procedures. *J Am Coll Cardiol*, 2016. 68(14): p. 1497–1504.
9. Maron BJ, Dearani JA, Ommen SR, et al. Low operative mortality achieved with surgical septal myectomy: Role of dedicated hypertrophic cardiomyopathy centers in the management of dynamic subaortic obstruction. *J Am Coll Cardiol*, 2015. 66(11): p. 1307–1308.
10. Panaich SS, Badheka AO, Chothani A, et al. Results of ventricular septal myectomy and hypertrophic cardiomyopathy (from nationwide inpatient sample [1998–2010]). *Am J Cardiol*, 2014. 114(9): p. 1390–1395.
11. Gersh BJ, Maron BJ, Bonow RO, et al. 2011 ACCF/AHA guideline for the diagnosis and treatment of hypertrophic cardiomyopathy: A report of the American College of Cardiology Foundation/American Heart Association Task Force on Practice Guidelines. *J Am Coll Cardiol*, 2011. 58(25): p. e212–e260.
12. Maron BJ, Nishimura RA. Surgical septal myectomy versus alcohol septal ablation: Assessing the status of the controversy in 2014. *Circulation*, 2014. 130(18): p. 1617–1624.
13. Mehaffey JH, Haywood NS, Hawkins RB, et al. Need for permanent pacemaker after surgical aortic valve replacement reduces long-term survival. *Ann Thorac Surg*, 2018. 106(2): p. 460–465.
14. McLeod CJ, Ommen SR, Ackerman MJ, et al. Surgical septal myectomy decreases the risk for appropriate implantable cardioverter defibrillator discharge in obstructive hypertrophic cardiomyopathy. *Eur Heart J*, 2007. 28(21): p. 2583–2588.

Chapter 10

VIRTUAL SURGICAL PLANNING FOR LEFT-VENTRICULAR MYECTOMY IN HYPERTROPHIC CARDIOMYOPATHY

Prahlad G. Menon and Srilakshmi M. Adhyapak

CONTENTS

INTRODUCTION

Hypertrophic cardiomyopathy (HCM), presenting with mid-ventricular obstruction and/or apical hypertrophy, is less common [1] than cases where obstruction is confined predominantly to the region of the left ventricular outflow tract (LVOT) [2]. Surgical resection of the hypertrophied myocardium has shown clinical benefit [2, 3]. However, incomplete resection may lead to recurrence, and excessive resection can lead to ventricular septal defects (VSD).

The traditional LVOT resection procedure, termed the classical Morrow procedure, has been associated with the recurrence of hypertrophic obstruction and therefore an extended myectomy has replaced the Morrow procedure [4]. In extended myectomy, the septal bulge is resected to the base of the papillary muscles. The revised myectomy extends well below the mitral valve tips and leaves a more even distribution of the septal thickness, and myectomy spares do not excise 3–5 mm below the aortic valve to avoid VSD and aortic regurgitation. The transaortic incision may have to be extended for this revised myectomy. Today, the extent of myectomy is guided predominantly by intra-operative palpation and visualization of the extent of sub-endocardial scar.

In HCM with mid-ventricular obstruction or apical hypertrophy, medical treatment has shown little benefit [5]. A proportion of these patients present with refractory heart failure and ventricular arrhythmias necessitating cardiac transplantation as a definitive surgery. Myectomy in these patients necessitates a ventriculotomy as the transaortic approach does not facilitate adequate exposure of the hypertrophied septum. Resection of the hypertrophied septum is predominantly guided by endocardial scar and intra-operative palpation [6]. The location of the papillary muscles as well as the location and extent of mid-ventricular obstruction is vital in guiding mid-ventricular and apical myectomy. Inadequate resection may lead to recurrence and apical aneurysm formation [6], whereas excessive resection can lead to VSD.

It is therefore paramount for the surgeon to precisely assess the pre-operative left ventricular (LV) anatomy prior to surgical intervention in the interest of optimizing adequate myectomy without damage to the surrounding structures. A pre-operative planning tool offering precise visualization of hypertrophic myocardial regions can aid in conducting more accurate surgical myectomy.

SURGICAL TECHNIQUE

Surgical myectomy is performed through standard median sternotomy. Typically, patients are started on a cardiopulmonary bypass by using direct aortic cannulation and a single two-stage venous cannula. Cold antegrade blood cardioplegia at 32 °C is used for myocardial protection. An apical ventriculotomy is made 2 to 2.5 cm lateral to the left anterior descending artery to avoid coronary compromise during closure of ventriculotomy. For mid-ventricular obstructions, the incision starts from the apex and is extended to the junction of the proximal two-third and distal one-third of the LV cavity medial, and to the base of the anterolateral papillary muscle. The papillary muscles and chordate are retracted laterally and the endocardial scar guides the section process. Using a combination of inspection and palpation, the thickened myocardium is identified and finally resection of the thickened myocardium is accomplished using a scalpel blade.

Left ventricular trabeculations are generally excised. If the anterolateral papillary muscle is hypertrophied, it is shaved evenly to facilitate blood flow in the mid-ventricle. Muscular resection adjacent to the ventriculotomy is limited so that excessive thinning of the edges does not complicate closure. After completing myectomy, the mitral valve apparatus is inspected to ensure that there has been no injury. Once the LV cavity has been well inspected, the ventriculotomy is closed. In one example, closure can be accomplished by buttressing with two Teflon strips using horizontal mattress sutures, which is followed over with additional mattress sutures with 2-0 Prolene.

In patients with additional LVOT obstruction, resection of the hypertrophied subaortic muscle is accomplished using a transaortic approach. However, the transaortic incision alone is not feasible for mid-ventricular myectomy as the obstruction is beyond surgical reach from the subaortic area. Ventriculotomy is generally not recommended to be extended to the subaortic region in order to avoid damage to the aortic valve and conduction system.

When pre-surgical planning is possible, the location as well as thickness/extent of myectomy is determined based on the areas where resection is needed, visually, by evaluating the pre-surgical plans (described in the next sections).

PRE-SURGICAL PLANNING

The LV endocardium and epicardium are reconstructed in three-dimensional (3D), cine steady-state free precession (SSFP) cardiac magnetic resonance (CMR) images, at each cardiac phase, starting with endocardial and epicardial contours demarcated at short-axis slices. As an example, this can be accomplished using Medviso Segment [7]. The pre-operative LV shape and function are quantified and the extent and location of hypertrophy in the mid-ventricular region was visualized at end-diastole. A pre-operative planning tool has been developed [8, 9] to first render these 3D myocardial surface reconstructions and simultaneously indicate the location and extent of regional hypertrophy within the LV cavity as a color map depicted on the endocardial surface, in the interest of guiding surgical myectomy. The tool is additionally capable of algorithmically and interactively deforming the endocardial surface in user-specified locations – simulative of myectomy – in the interest of facilitating optimal surgical resection of the hypertrophic myocardium.

In Menon et al. 2016 [8], virtual myectomy was performed on the LV in the end-diastolic phase, simulative of the likely shape of the LV in the cardioplegic state. Virtual myectomy was accomplished in 3D within an interactive pre-surgical planning software, using a free-form surface deformation tool applied to the endocardial surface at the hypertrophic regions.

Pre-operative LV volumes are quantified and the location as well as the extent of regional hypertrophy are visualized at the end-diastole cardiac phase using color maps of the myocardial wall thickness, prepared by quantifying the thickness enclosed between the endocardium and epicardium walls of the LV. Next, virtual myectomy is performed to resect the LV in the end-diastolic phase interactively using the VTK visualization environment. A free-form surface deformation tool is used to repeatedly morph and smooth the endocardial surface at hypertrophic regions in order to eliminate obstructive hypertrophic muscle, simulative of the real procedure. At each surgeon-selected location of virtual myectomy, the influence of an applied deformation as well as the magnitude of myectomy achieved is dictated using a Gaussian function. This function affects normally outward endocardial vertex movement and is controlled by means of a Gaussian amplitude coefficient and an influence coefficient defining the spatial territory around the point which is influenced by its deformation as a fraction of the Euclidean distance of an influenced endocardial vertex from the surgeon-specified site of myectomy. Poisson surface reconstruction is applied to the resulting endocardial point cloud after virtual surgical resection in order to effect a smooth surface for visualization. The following sub-sections illustrate the functioning of this tool in greater detail.

FREE-FORM VIRTUAL SURFACE DEFORMATION

The LV endocardium at end-diastole is developed into a set of uniformly spaced points and smoothly triangulated using a Poisson surface reconstruction approach to obtain a triangulated surface representation. At every point i on the triangulated endocardial surface, its Euclidean distance d_i to a specific position for virtual myectomy, selected by the surgeon, is computed. The surgeon is guided to this specific position based on 3D visualizations of the LV endocardium where hypertrophy is apparent based on the endocardial shape as well as the myocardial wall thickness, which was estimated visually based on a translucent rendering of the LV epicardial surface, superimposed on the endocardial surface model in our software. We denote the minimum value among d_i as d_{min}, that is:

$$d_{min} = \min\{d_i\} \tag{10.1}$$

A weighting factor was assigned to each point on the LV endocardium to functionally define the influence of an applied deformation from the surgeon-specific location for virtual myectomy, using a Gaussian function:

$$w_i = \alpha e^{(d_i - d_{min})/\beta} \tag{10.2}$$

where α is the amplitude coefficient of the Gaussian and β is the influence coefficient defining the spatial territory around the point which is influenced by its deformation. In our virtual myectomy procedures, α is set to 1 and β is a surgeon-defined parameter, set using an interactive slider bar in the graphical user interface of the software. Finally, each LV endocardial point was moved along its respective surface normal direction by the amount corresponding to its regional influence and amplitude factors, based on the surgeon-determined site for virtual myectomy. The moved position of a given point, P_{new}, is mathematically defined based on its pre-operative endocardial point position vector, P_{pre}, as:

$$P_{new} = P_{pre} + w_i \mathcal{N}\left(\sum_j n_j\right) \quad\quad (10.3)$$

where $\mathcal{N}(\cdot)$ is vector normalization operation applied to the normal vectors of each of the triangular facets, j, connected to a given point (i.e., n_j) in order to establish a mean normal direction of the triangular facets and therefore determine the directional movement of a given pre-operative endocardial point, P_{pre}.

In this manner, our interactive free-form deformation tool is designed to offer parametric control of the regional influence and magnitude of the myectomy in order to provide the surgeon with dexterous control for virtual correction of the LV shape. Regional color maps are prepared to visualize the precise location and extent (in mm units) of the virtual myectomy on the LV endocardium, in 3D.

Finally, the predicted post-operative LV shape is compared against 3D LV endocardial surface reconstructions at diastole, from post-operative CMR images obtained three months after surgery.

PRE-OPERATIVE PLANS FOR APICAL AND MID-VENTRICULAR OBSTRUCTION MYECTOMY – AN EXAMPLE

In pre-operative 3D reconstructions of the LV endocardium were analyzed for the distance of the mid-ventricular obstruction from the apex and the distance from the mitral annulus to the mid-ventricular obstruction, as well as the location and extent of hypertrophy based on a regional wall-thickness estimation process (see Figure 10.1). Figure 10.2 shows the result of surgical planning. Here the pre-operative LV cavity is represented as a green colored shell with the areas of hypertrophy that were virtually resected to reshape the LV endocardium colored in shades of red on the virtual post-operative model. The increasing red intensity signifies a greater magnitude of regional resection (in mm units).

Following virtual myectomy, there is a significant increase in the diastolic cavity size as measured by the LV end-diastolic volume. Further, under the assumption of an unchanged

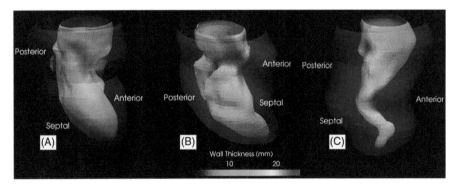

Figure 10.1 End-diastolic 3D renderings of the pre-operative LV endocardial surfaces in three representative patients (A,B,C) that are candidates for myectomy, illustrating the sites of mid-ventricular or apical hypertrophy as dents or depressions in the surface. All three illustrated patients had mid-ventricular hypertrophy as indicated by the indentations seen on the endocardial surfaces which correspond to regionally thicker myocardial walls (i.e., the space between the gray epicardial and the green endocardial surface). The patient illustrated in (C) additionally has apical hypertrophy. The regional wall thickness is color mapped from blue to green to red, indicative of increasing thickness (in mm units).

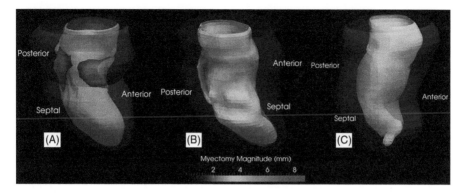

Figure 10.2 End-diastolic renderings of the virtual post-operative LV endocardial surfaces of the three patients (*A,B,C*) illustrated in Figure 10.2. The sites of virtual myectomy in the mid-ventricular or apical regions are color mapped from blue to red, indicative of the extent of the myectomy performed (in mm units).

end-systolic volume after myectomy, the virtual procedures additionally forecast a significant increase in the stroke volume.

During actual surgery, in the cardioplegic state, the LV is slightly lifted and displaced anteriorly and medially to the chest incision, to facilitate visual inspection of the LV cavity. Despite minor distortions in LV anatomy by this maneuver, it is still possible to identify the areas of hypertrophy demarcated in our patient-specific pre-operative plans, by using the left anterior descending coronary artery, the interventricular septum, the LV base, and the LV apex as landmarks.

IN VITRO PRE-SURGERY PRACTICE FOR OBSTRUCTIVE HCM

In this section, we describe surgical LV myectomy for patients with obstructive HCM in an *in vitro* setting. Here, rather than utilizing the 3D printed models as a basis for visualizing optimal surgical strategy, physical prototypes may be useful to actually practice the optimal surgical approach dictated by means of an image-based virtual pre-surgical planning step, prior to operating on the real patient. Three-dimensional prints of the LV chamber (factoring in the regional wall thickness) of patients with hypertrophy can be prepared with the goal of virtually resecting obstructions to blood flow out of the LV outflow tract, in the interest of facilitating optimal surgical myectomy through the experience of a pre-surgical performance with a full 3D field of view of the target anatomy (i.e., the LV).

However, while flexible materials for 3D printing are available and can be developed in various ways to have high or low regional stiffness, the latter is difficult to control and thermoplastic polymers (e.g., TPU filaments) are not always a good representation of tissue-specific constitutive material behaviors. Dermasol (DS-309, California Medical Innovations, Pomona CA) and Sylgard 184 are more feasible materials to prepare realistic physical models with more tissue-like constitutive material properties for the purpose of *in vitro* pre-surgical practice (see Figure 10.3), although they currently need to be utilized as a mold material, poured around a 3D printed core. As such, these materials can be molded in 3D printed mold shells, in order to prepare patient-specific models of the left ventricular myocardium, which in turn will be purposed for pre-surgical practice of the virtually planned patient-specific myectomy procedures.

Joshua Hermsen et al. [10] have studied the applications of 3D printing technology for surgical myectomy in HCM. 3D prints have been most commonly used as tangible adjuncts to the imaging modalities from which they are derived. These modalities are yet to attain a performable competence for clinical use. This study describes a process used for two patients undergoing septal myectomy for HCM. In Hermsen's study, the surgeon was provided with two tools: an interactive digital model and a physical 3D print. The digital model was a by-product of the

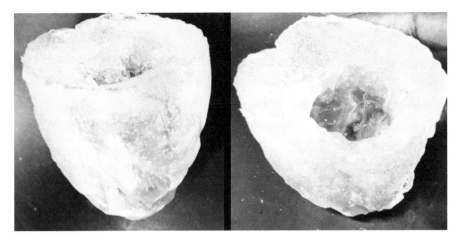

Figure 10.3 Molded LV myocardium model of a representative HCM patient, prepared out of Sylgard 184, by pouring and curing the material into a hollow patient-specific endocardial core bounded by an epicardial surface, for pre-surgical planning and practice of an ascertained computer-modeled myectomy strategy.

segmentation process necessary to create a 3D print from computed tomographic scan data, and was infinitely manipulable. The heart could be sectioned in any plane, and the image could be rotated on the screen in all axes. The ability to section, rotate, and view a 3D representation of the heart and ventricular septum in nontraditional planes as well as in sagittal, coronal, and axial planes was subjectively useful according to the assessment tool. The surgeon was also able to perform a virtual myectomy with the segmentation software. This was actually less useful than anticipated, however, because the graphical user interface for this function was not surgically intuitive. In addition, the volume of the digital resection was not calculable, so a comparison could not be made with the resection volumes from the 3D print and the patient.

The 3D-printed patient-specific model was sufficiently realistic in terms of operative exposure and anatomy. The overall assessment tool scores were modest. The model allowed realistic creation of the operative resection experience. In both patients tested, a dominant specimen was resected first and multiple smaller pieces were resected subsequently, just as is the usual practice in the operating room. Importantly, the 3D print allowed the performance of a more nearly ideal resection, because the print could be picked up, turned over, viewed and palpated from all angles, and resected further until the resultant septal anatomy appeared completely optimal. Because of its limitations, high costs, and lack of widespread applicability, how much this model would add to the depth of surgical experience in HCM of highly skilled and experienced cardiac surgeons is debatable.

VALIDATION OF THE PRE-OPERATIVE PLANNING TOOL

Three-dimensional virtual myectomy was performed on pre-operative hypertrophied LV endocardial surface reconstructions to visualize the likely post-operative LV shape after surgical myectomy in five patients [9]. Virtual outcomes were compared in 3D against true post-operative LV shapes in three patients, three months after surgery. The post-operative CMR-based endocardial reconstructions showed myectomy resections in the areas congruent with those predicted by means of pre-planning efforts, indicating that surgery was mostly implemented accurately as per the plans. In Figure 10.4, the pre-operatively prepared surgical plan is rendered translucently while the superimposed true post-operative rendering of the LV image is colored in solid green on the three representative patients with post-operative follow-up CMR studies. There was a significant decrease in LV mass following real myectomy. There was also an increase in the end-diastolic volume (EDV) and stroke volume (SV) following myectomy.

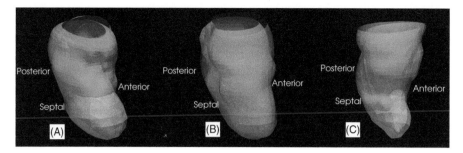

Figure 10.4 End-diastolic 3D renderings of the pre-operatively prepared surgical plan (rendered translucently) against the superimposed true post-operative rendering of the LV image (colored in solid green), for three patients (*A*,*B*,*C*) with post-operative follow-up CMR studies. Also shown for comparison with the surgical plans is the color mapped endocardial surfaces of each patient, representing regional myocardial wall thickness in the pre-operative LVs.

LIMITATIONS OF OUR PRE-SURGICAL PLANNING TOOL

Virtual myectomy may help in predicting EDV and SV which forms the basis for surgical myectomy. But pre-surgical planning does have limitations in guiding the extent of myectomy. At present, the magnitude of applied myectomy is largely selected based on the surgeon's judgment of the regional endocardial shape and wall thickness, as per 3D reconstructions from CMR images. However, surgeon guidance is imperative since myectomy should be avoided in the regions of compensatory hypertrophy of the lateral wall which are seen in the model. Further refinement of this technique is required to algorithmically determine the precise extent of thickness of the myocardium to be resected based on a collective estimation of normal myocardial wall-thickness estimates from a normal cohort. The latter may be feasible using machine learning methods and training on virtual surgical plans of myectomy procedures guided by surgeons.

In summary, pre-operative imaging using CMR can help facilitate quantification of pre-operative LV geometry for the location and magnitude of LV hypertrophy. Further, virtual myectomy has been demonstrated to be feasible using novel virtual surgical myectomy methods which help design a comprehensive strategy for myectomy, optimizing the precise location and extent of surgical myocardial resection, while preventing excessive resection or damage to adjacent ventricular structures. Incorporating our imaging-based virtual surgical approach as a standard pre-surgical planning tool has the potential to facilitate and guide precise and adequate myectomy in complex surgical procedures.

Finally, *in silico* methods for surgical planning can not only help pre-operatively visualize optimal cardiovascular remodeling, but can also aid in formulating an optimal palliative strategy for advanced heart failure. We introduce 3D printing and subsequent model molding to prepare patient-specific surgical templates, as an approach to further advance the virtual surgical planning pipeline, in the interest of *leveraging tactile interaction with physical anatomical prototypes for the purpose of pre-surgical practice, prior to operating on a real patient.*

REFERENCES

1. Cohen J, Effatt H, Goodwin JF, Oakley CM, Steiner RE. Hypertrophic obstructive cardiomyopathy. *Br Heart J.* 1964;26:16–32.
2. Gietzen H, Leuner C, Raute-Kreinsen U, Dellmann A, Hegselmann J, Strunk-Mueller C, et al. Acute and long-term results after transcoronary ablation of septal hypertrophy (TASH). Catheter interventional treatment for hypertrophic obstructive cardiomyopathy. *Eur Heart J.* 1999;1520:1342–1354.

3. Maron BJ, Bonow RO, Cannon RO III, Leon MB, Epstein SE. Hypertrophic cardiomyopathy. Interrelations of clinical manifestations, pathophysiology, and therapy. *N Engl J Med.* 1987;316:780–789.

4. Kunkala MR, Schaff HV, Nishimura RA, Abel MD, Sorajja P, Dearani JA. Transapical approach to myectomy for midventricular obstruction in hypertrophic cardiomyopathy. *Ann Thorac Surg.* 2013;96:564–570.

5. Sherrid MV, Chaudhry FA, Swistel DG. Obstructive hypertrophic cardiomyopathy: echocardiography, pathophysiology, and the continuing evolution of surgery for obstruction. *Ann Thorac Surg.* 2003;75:620–632.

6. Bonow RO, Carabello B, de Leon AC Jr, Edmunds LH Jr, Fedderly BJ, Freed MD, et al. Guidelines for the management of patients with valvular heart disease executive summary a report of the American College of Cardiology/American Heart Association Task Force on Practice Guidelines (Committee on Management of Patients With Valvular Heart Disease). *Circulation.*1998;98:1949–1984.

7. Heiberg E, Sjögren J, Ugander M, Carlsson M, Engblom H, Arheden H. Design and validation of Segment–freely available software for cardiovascular image analysis. *BMC Med Imaging.* 2010;10:1.

8. Menon PG, Rao PV, Adhyapak SM, Yuanchang O, Weeks R. Virtual surgical myectomy as a planning tool for obstructive hypertrophic cardiomyopathy. *J Cardiovasc Magn Reson.* 2016;18:P46.

9. Adhyapak SM, Menon PG, Rao Parachuri V. Improvements in left ventricular twist mechanics following myectomy for hypertrophic cardiomyopathy with mid-ventricular obstruction. *Inter Cardiovasc Thoracic Surgery.* 2017;25:128–130.

10. Hermsen JL, Burke TM, Seslar SP, Owens DS, Ripley BA, Mokadam NA, Verrier ED. Scan, plan, print, practice, perform: development and use of a patient-specific 3-dimensional printed model in adult cardiac surgery. *J Thorac Cardiovasc Surg.* 2016;153:132–140.

Chapter 11

ARRHYTHMIAS IN HYPERTROPHIC CARDIOMYOPATHY AND THEIR MANAGEMENT

Tom Kai Ming Wang and Milind Y. Desai

CONTENTS

INTRODUCTION

Hypertrophic cardiomyopathy (HCM) is defined by (a) the presence of $\geq$ 15 mm wall thickness in at least one left ventricular myocardial segment in adults and $\geq$ 2 standard deviations above the predicted mean in children on any form of cardiac imaging; and (b) findings that are not explained solely by loading conditions and that there is absence of HCM mimics such as amyloidosis and Fabry disease [1, 2]. Hypertrophic cardiomyopathy follows autosomal dominant inheritance with variable penetrance as a result of mutations in sarcomeric genes [3]. Alongside heart failure, left ventricular outflow tract (LVOT) obstruction, and angina, arrhythmias are an important clinical manifestation amongst the heterogeneous presentations of HCM. Arrhythmias can be classified as atrial tachyarrhythmias (especially atrial fibrillation [AF]), ventricular tachyarrhythmias, and bradyarrhythmias (including atrioventricular heart block [AVB]). Arrhythmias are extremely important because of their associated adverse cardiovascular events, especially sudden cardiac death (SCD), heart failure, stroke, and symptoms [2]. This chapter will outline the characteristics, risk factors, evaluation, and management of arrhythmias in HCM.

EPIDEMIOLOGY

Hypertrophic cardiomyopathy is the commonest form of hereditary heart disease, with a prevalence of 1 in 500 people [3]. Atrial fibrillation is the most prevalent sustained arrhythmia in both HCM and the general population, though it occurs at a four to six times higher rate in the former than the latter [4]. In a meta-analysis of 7,381 patients, the overall AF prevalence in HCM patients was 22.5%, and incidence was 3.1% per 100 patients per year [5]. Approximately two-thirds of AF is paroxysmal in HCM while the remainder are persistent or permanent [6]. Furthermore, a greater number of people have silent AF, at 24% in one study, which can then progress into symptomatic overt AF [7]. Other forms of atrial tachyarrhythmias, such as atrial flutter, atrial tachycardia, atrioventricular re-entrant tachycardia, and atrioventricular nodal re-entrant tachycardia, can all occur in HCM and share some of the clinical implications with AF [2].

Non-sustained ventricular tachycardia (NSVT) is often detected silently on monitoring, up to 31% in one study [8]. Ventricular tachyarrhythmias including ventricular tachycardia (VT) and ventricular fibrillation (VF) can both lead to SCD, which has decreased over time from 6% in earlier studies to a 1% annual incidence in contemporary studies with advances in HCM management [9, 10]. Apart from VT and VF, pulseless electrical activity, asystole, and AVB have all been reported with SCD in HCM [2].

Atrioventricular heart block is also rare in HCM, especially early on; however, those undergoing interventions to relieve LVOT obstruction such as septal myectomy and ablation are at especially high risk. Septal ablation has higher rates of pacemaker implantation for AVB than myectomy: 10% versus 4.4% respectively in one meta-analysis of 27 procedural cohorts and 4,804 patients [11]. Chronotropic incompetence is also not uncommon in HCM, reported at up to 50% in one study, and associated with reduced exercise tolerance [12].

PATHOPHYSIOLOGY

Many factors contribute to the abnormal structural and electrophysiological remodeling and development of atrial tachyarrhythmias in HCM. Left atrial afterload is increased by diastolic dysfunction from reduced left ventricular compliance and elevated filling pressures, as well as LVOT obstruction. Left atrial preload may also be increased by mitral regurgitation from systolic anterior motion of the mitral valve [13]. These can all lead to progressive left atrial dilation and remodeling that can alter its refractory period and provide a substrate for ectopy triggers [14]. At the histological level, myofibril disarray, fibrosis, ischemia, hypertrophy, and abnormal calcium handling in HCM have all been suggested to disturb intra-atrial conduction leading to AF [13]. There are also genetic factors, including the Arg663His missense mutation in the beta-myosin heavy chain seven gene and polymorphisms in the angiotensin receptor one gene associated with AF in HCM [15, 16].

A number of mechanisms have been proposed as the cause of ventricular tachyarrhythmias in HCM. The disarray of myocyte architecture in the ventricle correlates with hypertrophic segments in the ventricle, and demonstrates conduction delay, block, and decreased voltages [17]. Ischemia can occur when the heart muscle outgrows its coronary supply, as well as intramural vessels in thickened myocardium that remodel with luminal narrowing from wall hypertrophy. These processes can all contribute to myocardial fibrosis and necrosis [18]. It is suspected that VF originates mainly from the myofibril disarray segments while monomorphic VT predominantly from scar regions with re-entry [19]. Furthermore, sympathetic drive and tachycardias including sinus tachycardia and AF can also drive ventricular tachyarrhythmias in HCM, including in young patients and athletes.

As discussed earlier, septal ablation and myectomy patients are at high risk of AVB because of disturbance of the conducting system in close proximity to these interventions [11]. Atrioventricular-nodal blockers, particularly beta blockers that are indicated in many HCM patients with arrhythmias and/or LVOT obstruction, also can lead to AVB.

RISK FACTORS AND MULTI-MODALITY IMAGING

ATRIAL FIBRILLATION

Understanding the risk factors for arrhythmias in HCM is critical for stratification and prevention, and it is important to evaluate these clinically and with multi-modality imaging. Table 11.1 lists the risk factors for developing AF in HCM patients. Older age has been repeatedly shown to be associated with AF, for example, age > 50 years in one study, and > 40 years in another study, although AF can develop at all ages [6, 20–22]. Higher New York Heart Association (NYHA) class with heart failure predicts AF in some studies, as does female sex, hypertension, and vascular disease [6, 21, 22]. Features on electrocardiograms (ECGs) associated with AF in HCM include greater P-wave duration ($\geq$ 140 ms in one study) with signal averaging and P-wave dispersion ($\geq$ 52.5 ms) [23].

Multi-modality cardiac imaging, especially echocardiography and magnetic resonance imaging (MRI), plays a central role in the diagnosis of HCM, but also in reporting imaging factors associated with developing AF (Table 11.2) [1, 2]. One of the most important risk factors for developing AF in the general population, and also in HCM, is left atrial dimensions. One meta-analysis of 7,381 patients found a higher left atrial diameter in HCM patients with AF compared to sinus rhythm [5]. Left atrial volume index is a better marker of its size and remodeling than the current standard [24], and also predicts AF with increasing dilation [22, 25]. Left atrial measurements and emptying fraction (threshold < 38% in one study, which is a marker of left atrial dysfunction) are traditionally measured by echocardiography [24], but can also be assessed on MRI, and be prognostic of AF [20]. Significant mitral regurgitation, diastolic dysfunction parameters, and reduced left ventricular ejection fraction are also all associated with AF in HCM, but not in LVOT obstruction [22]. Furthermore, the degree of septal hypertrophy and presence of late gadolinium enhancement on MRI also appear to predict AF [14].

Table 11.1 Predictors for developing atrial fibrillation and thromboembolism in HCM

Atrial fibrillation in HCM	Thromboembolism in HCM [51]
Age > 40 or 50 years	Age, age/atrial fibrillation interaction
New York Heart Association class III-IV	New York Heart Association class III–IV
Left atrial diameter/left atrial volume index	Left atrial diameter
Vascular diseases	Vascular disease
Female sex	Atrial fibrillation
Hypertension	Prior thromboembolism
P-wave duration $\geq$ 140 ms	Maximal wall thickness (short axis)
P-wave dispersion $\geq$ 52.5 ms	
Left atrial emptying fraction	
Left ventricular ejection fraction	
Mitral regurgitation	
Diastolic dysfunction	
Late gadolinium enhancement	

Table 11.2 Echocardiography and MRI evaluation of HCM patients with arrhythmia or SCD risk

Echocardiography	MRI
Wall thickness and distribution	Wall thickness and distribution
Left ventricular dimensions (volume/mass)	Left ventricular dimensions (volume/mass)
Apical aneurysm	Apical aneurysm
Left ventricular ejection fraction	Left ventricular ejection fraction
Left ventricular global longitudinal strain	Left ventricular global longitudinal strain
Left atrial diameter/volume	Left atrial diameter/volume
Mitral anatomy/regurgitation/systolic anterior motion	Mitral regurgitation/systolic anterior motion
Left ventricular outflow tract peak velocity/ gradient	Left ventricular outflow tract peak velocity/gradient
Diastolic function	Late gadolinium enhancement

SUDDEN CARDIAC DEATH AND VENTRICULAR ARRHYTHMIAS

Most of the risk factors for SCD are well established and part of contemporary guidelines (Table 11.2) [1, 2]. The strongest risk factor is of course previous history of resuscitated cardiac arrest, VF, and sustained VT [26]. The other traditional risk factors are family history of SCD, unexplained syncope, increasing left ventricular hypertrophy, NSVT, and abnormal exercise blood pressure response [27, 28]. Family history of SCD is especially important in first-degree relatives, multiple family members, and in younger age relatives below 40–50 years old [29]. Unexplained syncope is common in about 20% of HCM, and may be a result of arrhythmia or LVOT obstruction; however, those occurring in the previous six months and younger patients confer the highest risk [30]. Non-sustained ventricular tachycardia is quite common and most prognostic in younger patients under 30 years old [27]. Nearly one-third of HCM patients have abnormal blood pressure response to exercise, whether from insufficient diastolic filling and therefore stroke volume and/or LVOT obstruction, and both predict SCD in younger patients while having a high negative predictive value > 95% [31]. Atrial fibrillation itself is associated with SCD as reported in a meta-analysis of 76,009 patients, including in HCM patients [32]. The relationship between age and SCD in HCM is complex as, although SCD is more common in younger patients, it occurs in all age groups [33]. Further research is also necessary to test whether genetic factors independently correlate with SCD risk when taking into account other clinical and imaging factors [34].

Echocardiography and MRI are also mandatory for SCD risk stratification. Increasing left ventricular wall thickness as a continuous parameter, and particularly when > 30 mm, predicts SCD [35]. Increasing left atrial diameter correlates with SCD risk [30]. Left ventricular outflow tract gradient, especially above ≥ 30 mm Hg, indicating obstruction, is also associated with SCD; however, it has a high negative predictive value of 96% but a low positive predictive value of 10% [36]. Several other imaging parameters reportedly associated with SCD are not yet part of contemporary guidelines. The presence of left ventricular systolic impairment (ejection fraction < 50%) is rare at 3.5% in one study and reflects end-stage HCM as another potential risk factor with high rates of defibrillator implantation at 10% per year [37]. Left ventricular global longitudinal strain has also been found to be associated with mortality and ventricular arrhythmias in HCM, including in a systematic review of 3,000 patients [38]. Apical aneurysms, which often involve extensive fibrosis, occur in a minority of apical HCM patients, which is about 2% and is therefore important to assess because of associations with SCD, strokes, and heart failure, especially when large at > 4 cm [39]. Late gadolinium enhancement on MRI is present in about two-thirds of HCM reflecting fibrosis, often within hypertrophied segments or at the right-ventricular hinge-points, have repeatedly been shown to be associated with SCD and all-cause mortality in HCM, including in a recent meta-analysis of 3,067 patients [40]. Multi-modality imaging therefore provides pivotal information for evaluating the risk of ventricular tachyarrhythmias and SCD in HCM patients to guide its management (Table 11.2) [41].

DIAGNOSIS AND MONITORING

The diagnosis of arrhythmias is based on ECG and rhythm monitoring. The latter includes findings from Holter monitors, implantable loop recorders, and cardiac implanted electronic devices (CIEDs), such as pacemakers and defibrillators. Atrial fibrillation is a supraventricular tachyarrhythmia with irregular R-R intervals, atrial activity, and absence of distinct repeat P-waves on ECG [42]. Ventricular tachycardia is the presence of at least three consecutive broad complexes originating from the ventricle at > 100 beats per minute, NSVT being < 30 seconds and sustained VT being ≥ 30 seconds [43]. Ventricular fibrillation shows rapid irregular electrical activity, usually > 300 bpm, with marked variability in electrocardiographic waveform. Sudden cardiac death is that thought to be a result of cardiac arrhythmia or hemodynamic catastrophe.

Conventional 12-lead ECG and 48-hour ambulatory ECG monitoring are both recommended on initial evaluation of suspected HCM to assist in its diagnosis [1, 2]. Both atrial and ventricular arrhythmias, non-sustained and sustained, can also be detected, which can help with the evaluation of symptoms and the risk of SCD and stroke at baseline. Furthermore, guidelines recommend regular monitoring in the follow-up on HCM patients, including annual ECGs at the time of clinical examination. Ambulatory electrocardiography to detect arrhythmias should be performed at the time of symptoms or regularly (Table 11.3). Both tests should also be performed within one to three months and at six to twelve months after invasive therapies to relieve LVOT obstruction. Echocardiography should be performed every one to two years, exercise testing every two to three years, and MRI every five years unless there is progressive disease.

Table 11.3 Summary of recommendations for atrial fibrillation management in HCM according to American and European guidelines with class and level of evidence

American 2011 guidelines [1]	European 2014 guidelines [2]
Monitoring	
• 24-hour ambulatory ECG monitoring for palpitations or light-headedness symptoms (IB) • 24-hour ambulatory ECG monitoring can be considered every 12 months for stable patients to evaluate atrial fibrillation (IIaC)	• 48-hour ambulatory ECG monitoring every 6–12 months to detect atrial fibrillation if LA diameter ≥ 45 mm, or with symptoms (IIaC)
Anticoagulation	
• Vitamin K antagonist anticoagulation INR 2.0–3.0 for atrial fibrillation (IC) • Non-vitamin K antagonist oral anticoagulants can be considered as alternative but data lacking (in 2011) • Left atrial appendage closure can be considered percutaneously or concurrently with cardiac surgery (IIaC)	• Lifelong vitamin K antagonist anticoagulation INR 2.0–3.0 unless contraindicated (IB) and flutter (IC) • Bleeding risk should be assessed (such as HAS-BLED score) when prescribing antithrombotic therapy (IIaB) • Non-vitamin K antagonist oral anticoagulants can be considered if failure to maintain therapeutic anticoagulation or side effects from vitamin K antagonists (IC) • Aspirin 75–100 mg plus clopidogrel 75 mg daily for patients who refuse oral anticoagulants (IIaB)

(Continued)

Table 11.3 (*Continued*) Summary of recommendations for atrial fibrillation management in HCM according to American and European guidelines with class and level of evidence

American 2011 guidelines [1]	European 2014 guidelines [2]
Rhythm control	
• Disopyramide (with rate-control agents) and amiodarone may be considered for rhythm control (IIaB) • Sotalol, dofetilide, and dronerdarone may be an alternative antiarrhythmic agent, especially in those with defibrillators (IIbC) • Catheter ablation can be performed in drug-refractory or intolerant atrial fibrillation (IIaB) • Surgical Maze procedure can be considered at time of cardiac surgery or in isolation (IIaC)	• Electrical or pharmacological (amiodarone) cardioversion for recent onset atrial fibrillation (IIaC) • Amiodarone to maintain sinus rhythm after cardioversion (IIaB) • Catheter ablation can be performed in drug-refractory or intolerant atrial fibrillation (IIaB)
Rate control	
• Beta blockers, verapamil, and diltiazem rate control for persistent or permanent atrial fibrillation (IC)	• Beta blockers, verapamil, and diltiazem rate control for persistent or permanent atrial fibrillation (IC) • Atrioventricular nodal ablation with pacemaker implantation (or cardiac resynchronization therapy pacemaker if left ventricular ejection fraction < 50%) for drug-refractory or intolerant permanent atrial fibrillation (IIbC)

MANAGEMENT

MEDICAL THERAPY FOR ARRHYTHMIAS

The management of AF in HCM patients is summarized in Table 11.3. Rate-control medications including beta blockers and non-dihydropyridine calcium channel blockers should be given to HCM patients with atrial arrhythmias, except when there is the presence of hemodynamic instability, acute heart failure, or pre-excitation [2]. These medications should also be used long term for AF whether paroxysmal or persistent to keep the resting heart rate at < 100 bpm while avoiding bradycardia [42]. Given that arrhythmias are poorly tolerated in HCM, rate-control medications should not defer a definitive plan for rhythm control in these patients. Beta blockers in particular are also used for ventricular arrhythmias and have separate important roles in the medical management of LVOT obstruction [1, 2].

Anti-arrhythmias like amiodarone can be considered for pharmacological rhythm control for acute AF especially with associated heart failure; however, if the patient is hemodynamically unstable, direct current cardioversion is preferred [2]. Electrical cardioversion can also be considered after at least three weeks of anticoagulation or with transesophageal echocardiography, which rules out intracardiac thrombus for rate-controlled AF. Pharmacological rhythm control strategies for other atrial tachyarrhythmias should follow contemporary guidelines [44]. Amiodarone and sotalol appear to suppress AF and supraventricular arrhythmias in observational studies long term, although there are no randomized trials [45, 46]. There is no data for dronerdarone and disopyramide (also used for LVOT obstruction) to suppress AF. Nevertheless amiodarone is often recommended for rhythm control long term, following AF cardioversion to sinus rhythm [2]. Both amiodarone and disopyramide have not reduced SCD in recent observational studies, although amiodarone is still sometimes used to suppress ventricular tachyarrhythmias if it is recurrent [47, 48].

ARRHYTHMIA ABLATION

Catheter ablation plays an important role in managing arrhythmias in the general population, with moderate efficacy for AF and ventricular arrhythmias, and high efficacy for other atrial tachyarrhythmias [42–44]. There is a strong need for rhythm control in HCM because of the adverse hemodynamic effects of tachycardia in these patients; however, anti-arrhythmics display weak if any evidence and also significant adverse effects, so their use should be minimized especially in younger patients. Recent studies have shown promise for catheter ablation in this setting but with some limitations, for example a meta-analysis of 386 patients with AF and HCM reported freedom from atrial arrhythmias, being 39% after 1 and 52% after > 1 procedures, which is lower than in patients without HCM, though adverse event rates were low [49]. The most important predictors of procedural success reported include smaller left atrial size, paroxysmal rather than persistent AF, younger age, lower NYHA class, shorter AF duration, and absence of LVOT obstruction. These are factors which may help in selecting patients for catheter ablation in HCM patients with AF. If AF is poorly controlled, despite pharmacological means, or is accompanied with significant side effects from drugs, then ablation of the atrioventricular node with pacemaker implantation may be considered (use a cardiac resynchronization therapy pacemaker if the left ventricular ejection fraction < 50%) [2]. Indications for ablation of all other supraventricular tachyarrhythmias should also follow contemporary guidelines and be strongly advocated [44]. Electrophysiological studies and ablation can also be considered for VT with focal origin, although current experience is restricted to small observational studies [50]. Further studies and trials are required to see if ablation reduces adverse cardiovascular events associated with atrial and ventricular arrhythmias in HCM patients.

THROMBOEMBOLISM PREVENTION

Atrial fibrillation is associated with higher risk of systemic thromboembolism in HCM patients, for example in a meta-analysis of 7,381 patients reporting rates of 3.8% per year and an overall 27.1% in HCM patients [5]. The predictors of thromboembolism in HCM have some differences compared to predictors for AF patients without HCM, with a large multi-center study finding age, previous thromboembolism, NYHA class, left atrial diameter, vascular disease, and maximal left ventricular wall thickness being associated with thromboembolic risk in HCM (Table 11.1) [51]. Anticoagulation is recommended by guidelines for HCM patients with AF, regardless of other risk factors, although bleeding risk should be assessed as well [2]. Vitamin K antagonists (VKA) are traditionally the first-line agents for thromboembolism prevention in selected VKA agents, with lower rates of stroke than antiplatelet agents [52]. More recently, a meta-analysis of 7,776 patients found non-VKA oral anticoagulants (NOACs) to have reduced risk of ischemic stroke, intracranial hemorrhage, and all-cause mortality compared to VKA, and similar rates of other embolic and bleeding events, suggesting NOACs are safe and effective alternatives to use in these patients [53]. Left atrial appendage closure at time of cardiac surgery, or percutaneously, may also be considered in selected patients [1].

IMPLANTABLE CARDIAC DEFIBRILLATORS

Avoidance of competitive sports is recommended in patients with HCM to prevent SCD [1, 2]. Implantable cardiac defibrillators (ICD) are a type of CIED and one of the cornerstones of HCM management for the effective primary and secondary prevention of SCD, with current guidelines summarized in Table 11.4 [1, 2, 54]. The indication is straightforward in secondary prevention of previously resuscitated cardiac arrest, syncope, or hemodynamic compromise from VT or VF with life expectancy of at least one year. For primary prevention, the risk evaluation is based on factors discussed in previous sections. The American guidelines suggest ICD as reasonable if HCM patients have family history of SCD in a first-degree relative, left ventricular wall thickness of at least 30 mm, or recent unexplained syncope, and may be

Table 11.4 Indications for ICDs in HCM by American and European guidelines and other risk factors

American 2011 guidelines [[(1)]	European 2014 guidelines [[(2)]
Indications	
• Prior cardiac arrest or sustained ventricular tachycardia (IB) • Family history of SCD in one or more first-degree relatives (IIaC) • Recent unexplained syncope (IIaC) • Left ventricular maximal wall thickness > 30 mm (IIaC) • Non-sustained ventricular tachycardia in presence of other SCD risk factors (IIaC); without these risk factors, usefulness of defibrillator uncertain (IIbC) • Abnormal blood pressure response with exercise in presence of other SCD risk factors (IIaC); without these risk factors, usefulness of defibrillator uncertain (IIbC) • High risk children with unexplained syncope, massive left ventricular hypertrophy, or family history of SCD taking into account high complication rates of long-term defibrillator (IIaC)	• Prior cardiac arrest from ventricular tachycardia or fibrillation, or sustained ventricular tachycardia causing syncope or hemodynamic compromise, and life expectancy > 1 year (IB) • HCM Risk-SCD calculator is recommended to estimate five-year risk of SCD for primary prevention in patients ≥ 16 years old (IB) • HCM Risk-SCD five-year risk ≥ 6% and life expectancy > 1 year following detailed clinical assessment (IIaB) • HCM Risk-SCD five-year risk ≥ 4–6% and life expectancy > 1 year may be considered following detailed clinical assessment (IIbB)
Contraindications	
• Routine implantation in patients without above indications (IIIC) • To allow patients to participate in competitive sports(IIIC) • Genotype positive but phenotype negative patients	• HCM Risk-SCD five-year risk < 4% and no other risk factors (IIIB)

considered for non-sustained VT or abnormal blood pressure response with exercise [1]. The European guidelines utilize the HCM Risk-SCD calculator based on age, family history of SCD, unexplained syncope, LVOT gradient, left ventricular maximum wall thickness, left atrial diameter, and NSVT [2, 28]. Intracardiac defibrillator is indicated if the five-year calculated risk of SCD is ≥ 6% and can be considered if 4–6%. This should be assessed at baseline, every one to two years, and when there is a change in clinical status.

Other considerations are necessary prior to and after ICD implantation [2]. Patients need counseling regarding the complications of ICD, especially inappropriate shocks, as well as restrictions on driving, occupational, and other activities. Subcutaneous ICDs are now an alternative to transvenous systems in appropriate HCM patients without indications for pacing. Anti-tachycardia pacing may help terminating VT. The ICD's VF shock zone should be set above 220/minute to prevent shocks from AF with rapid conduction. Device interrogation needs to be thorough, distinguishing supraventricular and ventricular arrhythmias, and may require device reprogramming. Options to consider in those with recurrent shocks and ventricular arrhythmias include beta-blockers, amiodarone, and electrophysiology study with catheter ablation as necessary.

PACING

It is important to reduce or remove pharmacological agents that slow the heart rate if HCM patients present with bradycardias and/or AVB. Also, extra care needs to be taken when managing patients who have had invasive interventions to relieve LVOT obstruction because of their elevated risk of AVB [11]. Otherwise, the indications for pacing should follow contemporary guidelines [55]. Pacemaker implantation is also necessary if atrioventricular nodal ablation is performed for drug-refractory AF rate control (dual-chamber if paroxysmal AF, single-chamber if permanent) [2]. Furthermore, cardiac resynchronization therapy should be considered in those with reduced ejection fraction, along with other conventional criteria of left bundle branch block, QRS > 120 ms and heart failure symptoms despite optimal medical therapy [55]. Such devices often incorporate defibrillating functions in HCM patients to offer protection from bradycardias, ventricular arrhythmias, SCD, and heart failure.

CONCLUSION

Arrhythmias are commonly encountered in HCM, particularly AF and ventricular arrhythmias, and are associated with adverse cardiovascular events including SCD, heart failure, and stroke. Key and often common risk factors exist for atrial and ventricular tachyarrhythmias that require regular and thorough clinical, arrhythmia, and multi-modality imaging evaluation. There are multiple facets to the management of arrhythmias in HCM, including medical therapies for arrhythmias, anticoagulation, ablation, and CIEDs. Clinicians need to have a sound understanding of these management strategies in order to optimize outcomes in HCM patients.

REFERENCES

1. Gersh BJ, Maron BJ, Bonow RO, Dearani JA, Fifer MA, Link MS, et al. 2011 ACCF/AHA guideline for the diagnosis and treatment of hypertrophic cardiomyopathy: a report of the American College of Cardiology Foundation/American Heart Association Task Force on Practice Guidelines – developed in collaboration with the American Association for Thoracic Surgery, American Society of Echocardiography, American Society of Nuclear Cardiology, Heart Failure Society of America, Heart Rhythm Society, Society for Cardiovascular Angiography and Interventions, and Society of Thoracic Surgeons. *Journal of the American College of Cardiology.* 2011 Dec 13;58(25):e212–e260.

2. Elliott PM, Anastasakis A, Borger MA, Borggrefe M, Cecchi F, Charron P, et al. 2014 ESC guidelines on diagnosis and management of hypertrophic cardiomyopathy: the Task Force for the Diagnosis and Management of Hypertrophic Cardiomyopathy of the European Society of Cardiology (ESC). *European Heart Journal.* 2014 Oct 14;35(39):2733–2779.

3. Maron BJ, Maron MS. Hypertrophic cardiomyopathy. *Lancet.* 2013 Jan 19;381 (9862):242–255.

4. MacIntyre C, Lakdawala NK. Management of atrial fibrillation in hypertrophic cardiomyopathy. *Circulation.* 2016 May 10;133(19):1901–1905.

5. Guttmann OP, Rahman MS, O'Mahony C, Anastasakis A, Elliott PM. Atrial fibrillation and thromboembolism in patients with hypertrophic cardiomyopathy: systematic review. *Heart.* 2014 Mar;100(6):465–472.

6. Olivotto I, Cecchi F, Casey SA, Dolara A, Traverse JH, Maron BJ. Impact of atrial fibrillation on the clinical course of hypertrophic cardiomyopathy. *Circulation.* 2001 Nov 20;104(21):2517–2524.

7. Rowin EJ, Orfanos A, Estes NAM, Wang W, Link MS, Maron MS, et al. Occurrence and natural history of clinically silent episodes of atrial fibrillation in hypertrophic cardiomyopathy. *The American Journal of Cardiology.* 2017 Jun 1;119(11):1862–1865.

8. Adabag AS, Casey SA, Kuskowski MA, Zenovich AG, Maron BJ. Spectrum and prognostic significance of arrhythmias on ambulatory Holter electrocardiogram in hypertrophic cardiomyopathy. *Journal of the American College of Cardiology.* 2005 Mar 1;45(5):697–704.

9. Hardarson T, De la Calzada CS, Curiel R, Goodwin JF. Prognosis and mortality of hypertrophic obstructive cardiomyopathy. *Lancet.* 1973 Dec 29;2(7844):1462–1467.

10. Elliott PM, Gimeno JR, Thaman R, Shah J, Ward D, Dickie S, et al. Historical trends in reported survival rates in patients with hypertrophic cardiomyopathy. *Heart.* 2006 Jun;92(6):785–791.

11. Liebregts M, Vriesendorp PA, Mahmoodi BK, Schinkel AF, Michels M, ten Berg JM. A systematic review and meta-analysis of long-term outcomes after septal reduction therapy in patients with hypertrophic cardiomyopathy. *JACC Heart Failure.* 2015 Nov;3(11):896–905.

12. Efthimiadis GK, Giannakoulas G, Parcharidou DG, Pagourelias ED, Kouidi EJ, Spanos G, et al. Chronotropic incompetence and its relation to exercise intolerance in hypertrophic cardiomyopathy. *International Journal of Cardiology.* 2011 Dec 1;153(2):179–184.

13. Garg L, Gupta M, Sabzwari SRA, Agrawal S, Agarwal M, Nazir T, et al. Atrial fibrillation in hypertrophic cardiomyopathy: prevalence, clinical impact, and management. *Heart Failure Reviews.* 2019 Mar;24(2):189–197.

14. Papavassiliu T, Germans T, Fluchter S, Doesch C, Suriyakamar A, Haghi D, et al. CMR findings in patients with hypertrophic cardiomyopathy and atrial fibrillation. *Journal of Cardiovascular Magnetic Resonance.* 2009 Sep 9;11:34.

15. Gruver EJ, Fatkin D, Dodds GA, Kisslo J, Maron BJ, Seidman JG, et al. Familial hypertrophic cardiomyopathy and atrial fibrillation caused by Arg663His beta-cardiac myosin heavy chain mutation. *The American Journal of Cardiology.* 1999 Jun 17;83(12a):13h–18h.

16. Tuluce K, Tuluce SY. Predictors of atrial fibrillation risk in hypertrophic cardiomyopathy. *Journal of Atrial Fibrillation.* 2015 Feb–Mar;7(5):1200.

17. Schumacher B, Gietzen FH, Neuser H, Schummelfeder J, Schneider M, Kerber S, et al. Electrophysiological characteristics of septal hypertrophy in patients with hypertrophic obstructive cardiomyopathy and moderate to severe symptoms. *Circulation.* 2005 Oct 4;112(14):2096–2101.

18. Moore B, Semsarian C, Chan KH, Sy RW. Sudden cardiac death and ventricular arrhythmias in hypertrophic cardiomyopathy. *Heart, Lung & Circulation.* 2019 Jan;28(1):146–154.

19. Cha YM, Gersh BJ, Maron BJ, Boriani G, Spirito P, Hodge DO, et al. Electrophysiologic manifestations of ventricular tachyarrhythmias provoking appropriate defibrillator interventions in high-risk patients with hypertrophic cardiomyopathy. *Journal of Cardiovascular Electrophysiology.* 2007 May;18(5):483–487.

20. Maron BJ, Haas TS, Maron MS, Lesser JR, Browning JA, Chan RH, et al. Left atrial remodeling in hypertrophic cardiomyopathy and susceptibility markers for atrial fibrillation identified by cardiovascular magnetic resonance. *The American Journal of Cardiology.* 2014 Apr 15;113(8):1394–1400.

21. Guttmann OP, Pavlou M, O'Mahony C, Monserrat L, Anastasakis A, Rapezzi C, et al. Predictors of atrial fibrillation in hypertrophic cardiomyopathy. *Heart.* 2017 May;103(9):672–678.

22. Siontis KC, Geske JB, Ong K, Nishimura RA, Ommen SR, Gersh BJ. Atrial fibrillation in hypertrophic cardiomyopathy: prevalence, clinical correlations, and mortality in a large high-risk population. *Journal of the American Heart Association.* 2014 Jun 25;3(3):e001002.

23. Ozdemir O, Soylu M, Demir AD, Topaloglu S, Alyan O, Turhan H, et al. P-wave durations as a predictor for atrial fibrillation development in patients with hypertrophic cardiomyopathy. *International Journal of Cardiology.* 2004 Apr;94(2–3):163–166.

24. Lang RM, Badano LP, Mor-Avi V, Afilalo J, Armstrong A, Ernande L, et al. Recommendations for cardiac chamber quantification by echocardiography in adults: an update from the American Society of Echocardiography and the European Association of Cardiovascular Imaging. *Journal of the American Society of Echocardiography.* 2015 Jan;28(1):1–39.e14.

25. Tani T, Tanabe K, Ono M, Yamaguchi K, Okada M, Sumida T, et al. Left atrial volume and the risk of paroxysmal atrial fibrillation in patients with hypertrophic cardiomyopathy. *Journal of the American Society of Echocardiography.* 2004 Jun;17(6):644–648.

26. Elliott PM, Sharma S, Varnava A, Poloniecki J, Rowland E, McKenna WJ. Survival after cardiac arrest or sustained ventricular tachycardia in patients with hypertrophic cardiomyopathy. *Journal of the American College of Cardiology.* 1999 May;33(6):1596–1601.

27. Christiaans I, van Engelen K, van Langen IM, Birnie E, Bonsel GJ, Elliott PM, et al. Risk stratification for sudden cardiac death in hypertrophic cardiomyopathy: systematic review of clinical risk markers. *Europace: European Pacing, Arrhythmias, and Cardiac Electrophysiology* 2010 Mar;12(3):313–321.

28. O'Mahony C, Jichi F, Pavlou M, Monserrat L, Anastasakis A, Rapezzi C, et al. A novel clinical risk prediction model for sudden cardiac death in hypertrophic cardiomyopathy (HCM risk-SCD). *European Heart Journal.* 2014 Aug 7;35(30):2010–2020.

29. Maron MS. Family history of sudden death should be a primary indication for implantable cardioverter defibrillator in hypertrophic cardiomyopathy. *The Canadian Journal of Cardiology.* 2015 Nov;31(11):1402–1406.

30. Spirito P, Autore C, Rapezzi C, Bernabo P, Badagliacca R, Maron MS, et al. Syncope and risk of sudden death in hypertrophic cardiomyopathy. *Circulation.* 2009 Apr 7;119(13):1703–1710.

31. Olivotto I, Maron BJ, Montereggi A, Mazzuoli F, Dolara A, Cecchi F. Prognostic value of systemic blood pressure response during exercise in a community-based patient population with hypertrophic cardiomyopathy. *Journal of the American College of Cardiology.* 1999 Jun;33(7):2044–2051.

32. Rattanawong P, Upala S, Riangwiwat T, Jaruvongvanich V, Sanguankeo A, Vutthikraivit W, et al. Atrial fibrillation is associated with sudden cardiac death: a systematic review and meta-analysis. *Journal of Interventional Cardiac Electrophysiology.* 2018 Mar;51(2):91–104.

33. Maron BJ, Olivotto I, Spirito P, Casey SA, Bellone P, Gohman TE, et al. Epidemiology of hypertrophic cardiomyopathy-related death: revisited in a large non-referral-based patient population. *Circulation.* 2000 Aug 22;102(8):858–864.

34. Weissler-Snir A, Adler A, Williams L, Gruner C, Rakowski H. Prevention of sudden death in hypertrophic cardiomyopathy: bridging the gaps in knowledge. *European Heart Journal.* 2017 Jun 7;38(22):1728–1737.

35. Spirito P, Bellone P, Harris KM, Bernabo P, Bruzzi P, Maron BJ. Magnitude of left ventricular hypertrophy and risk of sudden death in hypertrophic cardiomyopathy. *The New England Journal of Medicine.* 2000 Jun 15;342(24):1778–1785.

36. Elliott P, Gimeno J, Tome M, McKenna W. Left ventricular outflow tract obstruction and sudden death in hypertrophic cardiomyopathy. *European Heart Journal.* 2006 Dec;27(24):3073; author reply-4.

37. Harris KM, Spirito P, Maron MS, Zenovich AG, Formisano F, Lesser JR, et al. Prevalence, clinical profile, and significance of left ventricular remodeling in the end-stage phase of hypertrophic cardiomyopathy. *Circulation.* 2006 Jul 18;114(3):216–225.

38. Tower-Rader A, Mohananey D, To A, Lever HM, Popovic ZB, Desai MY. Prognostic value of global longitudinal strain in hypertrophic cardiomyopathy: a systematic review of existing literature. *JACC Cardiovascular Imaging.* 2019 Oct;12(10):1930–1942.

39. Maron MS, Finley JJ, Bos JM, Hauser TH, Manning WJ, Haas TS, et al. Prevalence, clinical significance, and natural history of left ventricular apical aneurysms in hypertrophic cardiomyopathy. *Circulation.* 2008 Oct 7;118(15):1541–1549.

40. Briasoulis A, Mallikethi-Reddy S, Palla M, Alesh I, Afonso L. Myocardial fibrosis on cardiac magnetic resonance and cardiac outcomes in hypertrophic cardiomyopathy: a meta-analysis. *Heart.* 2015 Sep;101(17):1406–1411.

41. Cardim N, Galderisi M, Edvardsen T, Plein S, Popescu BA, D'Andrea A, et al. Role of multimodality cardiac imaging in the management of patients with hypertrophic cardiomyopathy: an expert consensus of the European Association of Cardiovascular Imaging Endorsed by the Saudi Heart Association. *European Heart Journal Cardiovascular Imaging.* 2015 Mar;16(3):280.

42. January CT, Wann LS, Alpert JS, Calkins H, Cigarroa JE, Cleveland JC, Jr., et al. 2014 AHA/ACC/HRS guideline for the management of patients with atrial fibrillation: a report of the American College of Cardiology/American Heart Association Task Force on Practice Guidelines and the Heart Rhythm Society. *Journal of the American College of Cardiology.* 2014 Dec 2;64(21):e1–76.

43. Al-Khatib SM, Stevenson WG, Ackerman MJ, Bryant WJ, Callans DJ, Curtis AB, et al. 2017 AHA/ACC/HRS guideline for management of patients with ventricular arrhythmias and the prevention of sudden cardiac death: a report of the American College of Cardiology/American Heart Association Task Force on Clinical Practice Guidelines and the Heart Rhythm Society. *Journal of the American College of Cardiology.* 2018 Oct 2;72(14):e91–220.

44. Page RL, Joglar JA, Caldwell MA, Calkins H, Conti JB, Deal BJ, et al. 2015 ACC/AHA/HRS guideline for the management of adult patients with supraventricular tachycardia: a report of the American College of Cardiology/American Heart Association Task Force on Clinical Practice Guidelines and the Heart Rhythm Society. *Journal of the American College of Cardiology.* 2016 Apr 5;67(13):e27–115.

45. Robinson K, Frenneaux MP, Stockins B, Karatasakis G, Poloniecki JD, McKenna WJ. Atrial fibrillation in hypertrophic cardiomyopathy: a longitudinal study. *Journal of the American College of Cardiology.* 1990 May;15(6):1279–1285.

46. Tendera M, Wycisk A, Schneeweiss A, Polonski L, Wodniecki J. Effect of sotalol on arrhythmias and exercise tolerance in patients with hypertrophic cardiomyopathy. *Cardiology.* 1993;82(5):335–342.

47. Melacini P, Maron BJ, Bobbo F, Basso C, Tokajuk B, Zucchetto M, et al. Evidence that pharmacological strategies lack efficacy for the prevention of sudden death in hypertrophic cardiomyopathy. *Heart.* 2007 Jun;93(6):708–710.

48. Sherrid MV, Barac I, McKenna WJ, Elliott PM, Dickie S, Chojnowska L, et al. Multicenter study of the efficacy and safety of disopyramide in obstructive hypertrophic cardiomyopathy. *Journal of the American College of Cardiology.* 2005 Apr 19;45(8):1251–1258.

49. Providencia R, Elliott P, Patel K, McCready J, Babu G, Srinivasan N, et al. Catheter ablation for atrial fibrillation in hypertrophic cardiomyopathy: a systematic review and meta-analysis. *Heart.* 2016 Oct 1;102(19):1533–1543.

50. Dukkipati SR, d'Avila A, Soejima K, Bala R, Inada K, Singh S, et al. Long-term outcomes of combined epicardial and endocardial ablation of monomorphic ventricular tachycardia related to hypertrophic cardiomyopathy. *Circulation Arrhythmia and Electrophysiology.* 2011 Apr;4(2):185–194.

51. Guttmann OP, Pavlou M, O'Mahony C, Monserrat L, Anastasakis A, Rapezzi C, et al. Prediction of thrombo-embolic risk in patients with hypertrophic cardiomyopathy (HCM Risk-CVA). *European Journal of Heart Failure.* 2015 Aug;17(8):837–845.

52. Maron BJ, Olivotto I, Bellone P, Conte MR, Cecchi F, Flygenring BP, et al. Clinical profile of stroke in 900 patients with hypertrophic cardiomyopathy. *Journal of the American College of Cardiology.* 2002 Jan 16;39(2):301–307.

53. Zhou Y, He W, Zhou Y, Zhu W. Non-vitamin K antagonist oral anticoagulants in patients with hypertrophic cardiomyopathy and atrial fibrillation: a systematic review and meta-analysis. *Journal of Thrombosis and Thrombolysis.* 2019 Dec 2.

54. Maron BJ, Spirito P, Shen WK, Haas TS, Formisano F, Link MS, et al. Implantable cardioverter-defibrillators and prevention of sudden cardiac death in hypertrophic cardiomyopathy. *Jama.* 2007 Jul 25;298(4):405–412.

55. Kusumoto FM, Schoenfeld MH, Barrett C, Edgerton JR, Ellenbogen KA, Gold MR, et al. 2018 ACC/AHA/HRS guideline on the evaluation and management of patients with bradycardia and cardiac conduction delay: A report of the American College of Cardiology/American Heart Association Task Force on Clinical Practice Guidelines and the Heart Rhythm Society. *Journal of the American College of Cardiology.* 2019 Aug 20;74(7):e51–156.

Chapter 12

PERCUTANEOUS TRANSLUMINAL SEPTAL MYOCARDIAL ABLATION IN HYPERTROPHIC CARDIOMYOPATHY

Anene C. Ukaigwe and Paul Sorajja

CONTENTS

INTRODUCTION

Hypertrophic cardiomyopathy (HCM) is an inherited cardiac disease estimated from echocardiographic studies to affect 1 in 500 persons [1]. From gene-based studies, the prevalence may be 1 in 200 [2]. The gene mutations result in abnormal coding of sarcomeric proteins which are inherited in an autosomal dominant Mendelian fashion with variable penetrance. Mutations manifest phenotypically as left ventricular hypertrophy in the absence of other causes diagnosed on echocardiograms or cardiac magnetic resonance imaging (CMR).

Dynamic left ventricular outflow tract obstruction (LVOTO) in HCM results from a complex interaction between the effects of left ventricular septal hypertrophy as well as Venturi and drag forces in the left ventricular outflow tract (LVOT), causing systolic anterior motion (SAM) of the mitral valve. Left ventricular hypertrophy reduces the area of the LVOT and SAM obstructs flow in the LVOT due to SAM–septal contact. Both of these lead to LVOTO and left ventricular hypertension. Mitral valve abnormalities (a long anterior mitral leaflet, anterior and inward displacement of the papillary muscles) are frequently associated with HCM and contribute to dynamic LVOTO. Systolic anterior motion also results in malcoaptation of the mitral valve, causing posteriorly directed mitral regurgitation. Left ventricular outflow tract obstruction, LV hypertension, and mitral regurgitation lead to elevated left atrial and ventricular pressure as well as reduced cardiac output, which manifests as heart failure symptoms.

Dynamic LVOTO can be found in 30% of HCM patients at rest and 30% elicited with provocative measures [3]. Dynamic LVOTO presents a wide range of symptoms, making clear clinical stratification challenging. For those with lifestyle-limiting symptoms, negative inotropic agents (beta blockers, non-dihydropyridine calcium channel blockers, and disopyramide) are effective first-line therapies. When symptoms attributable to dynamic LVOTO persist, despite maximally tolerated medical therapy or when side effects limit medical therapy, then septal reduction therapy (SRT) with surgical myectomy or percutaneous options are indicated.

Percutaneous transluminal septal myocardial ablation (PTSMA) refers to percutaneous SRT alternatives to surgical septal myectomy that address LVOTO, defined as an LVOT gradient of 30 mm Hg at rest or 50 mm Hg with provocation. The first successful PTSMA, alcohol septal ablation (ASA), was first reported by Ulrich Sigwart in 1995, in which alcohol injection through one or more septal branches caused a controlled localized basal septal infarction and relieved dynamic LVOTO [4]. Since then, the procedure has been rapidly adopted and has emerged as an effective SRT to alleviate obstructive symptoms of HCM.

SEPTAL REDUCTION THERAPIES

The technical goal of SRTs is reducing the systolic thickening of the interventricular septum that results in mechanical obstruction as well as SAM of the mitral valve – both of which cause LVOTO and mitral regurgitation. In appropriately selected patients who have obstructive symptoms of HCM, SRT improves functional status and quality of life. Ideally, while the impact on survival remains debatable, SRT should normalize the survival of HCM patients to comparable-age and gender-matched controls while minimizing procedural mortality and the risk of sudden cardiac death, as suggested in several clinical registries.

Surgical myectomy is a complex procedure that involves resection of muscle at the basal septum [5]. Since its initial description by Morrow in 1975, the procedure has evolved to include extended myectomy, and papillary and mitral valve surgery to enhance its benefits. Myectomy is effective at abolishing LVOTO and mitral regurgitation which in turn normalize left ventricular and left atrial pressures as well as heart failure symptoms. At the same time, other diseases can be treated surgically, for example, valve disease and coronary artery disease. The operative mortality for isolated myectomy is < 1% in experienced centers [6]. Real-world experience obtained from the US Nationwide Inpatient Sample evaluated outcomes of SRT in US hospitals [7]. The volumes of each center were stratified into tertiles. This study showed that the volume of myectomy in most centers was very low (a median of one procedure per year). A volume–outcome relationship was demonstrated, showing superior outcomes in large volume centers. Peri-procedural mortality in the high-volume tertile centers (3.8%) in this study surpassed outcomes in specialized HCM centers where mortality was < 1% [8]. This emphasizes the benefits of multidisciplinary care [7, 9, 10]. The European Society of Cardiology (ESC) 2014 HCM guidelines recommend a minimum annual volume of ten septal myectomies per operator, and each program should have at least two myectomy surgeons, though this is not based on outcome data [11]. The American College of Cardiology guidelines for the diagnosis and management of HCM recommend that myectomy operators perform at least 20 procedures or work within a program that has performed at least 50 procedures with the goals of < 1% operative mortality and < 3% major morbidity [12].

The paucity of experienced centers as well as longer recovery times make myectomy less accessible and enhance the need for less invasive and readily available SRTs. Since the initial PTSMA in 1994, it has evolved to become the predominant SRT in Europe [13]. With increasing experience and long-term outcomes, PTSMA has emerged as a class I indication similar to myectomy in the European guidelines in adult patients who do not require additional cardiac surgical procedures.

Percutaneous transluminal septal myocardial ablation uses angiographic and echocardiographic guidance and standard percutaneous coronary intervention techniques to cause a controlled infarction at the basal septum. The resulting septal hypokinesis and paradoxical septal motion reduce LVOTO and SAM, with these effects continuing for several weeks as remodeling from the infarct progresses. Percutaneous transluminal septal myocardial ablation significantly improves symptoms without decreasing survival [14]. However, it is associated with a relatively higher risk of permanent pacemaker requirement, is reliant on an inflexible septal anatomy, and may not address associated abnormalities common in HCM, such as anterior papillary muscle displacement as well as intrinsic mitral valve disease.

As with any therapy, the choice between surgical or percutaneous SRT requires careful consideration of operator expertise, procedural risk, institutional outcomes, and comorbidities. This is best made within the context of a multidisciplinary heart team in a comprehensive HCM center.

PATIENT SELECTION AND PRE-PROCEDURAL ASSESSMENT

Percutaneous transluminal septal myocardial ablation is indicated for patients who have:

1   Angina, dyspnea (NYHA III/IV) or exertional syncope or presyncope refractory to medical therapy or intolerance to medical therapy;

2   A dynamic LVOTO (LVOT gradient ≥ 30 mm Hg at rest or ≥ 50 mm Hg with provocation) due to SAM of the mitral valve in the absence of intrinsic mitral valve disease;

3   A targeted septal thickness sufficient to perform the procedure safely and effectively in the judgment of the operator, typically with ventricular septal thickness ≥ 15 mm, ≤ 26 mm;

4   No need for cardiac surgery (e.g., due to left main or multivessel coronary artery disease, valve replacement, subaortic membrane, anomalous papillary muscles);

5   A suitable septal branch supplying the basal septum involved in LVOT obstruction.

The presence of dynamic LVOTO is measured by peak-to-peak gradients on invasive hemodynamics or peak LVOT gradients on a Doppler echocardiogram. Mid-cavitary obstruction and fixed LVOTO due to a subaortic membrane have to be excluded by echocardiogram or invasive hemodynamics as ASA does not adequately address this. The Doppler envelop of dynamic LVOTO must be carefully distinguished from that of mitral regurgitation which can be challenging due to the proximity and the systolic timing of both. Systolic anterior motion of the mitral valve associated with dynamic LVOTO should also be assessed by echocardiogram. Mitral regurgitation that accompanies SAM is posteriorly directed, therefore any other direction of the mitral regurgitant jet suggests intrinsic mitral valve disease, which cannot be effectively addressed by PTSMA, in which case mitral valve repair is needed. This has traditionally been surgical repair, but recent experience shows that, in carefully selected patients, percutaneous Mitraclip (Abbott Vascular, CA) therapy can be successfully employed to plicate the SAM of the mitral valve, treat mitral regurgitation as well as reduce dynamic LVOTO [15].

Septal wall thickness should be assessed and PTSMA should only be performed if the former is felt to be favorable by the operator. A thin septal wall (i.e., < 15 mm) carries a risk of ventricular septal defect. In these patients, mitral valve repair or plication should be considered. Septal wall thickness of > 25 mm requires larger amounts of alcohol for effective ablation, and there is the potential for the development of extensive scarring and a higher risk of arrhythmias [16]. Percutaneous transluminal septal myocardial ablation in a thick septum of > 30 mm is also associated with worse long-term outcomes [17], which may be due to inadequate gradient reduction, the need for large volumes of alcohol, and scar formation to reduce LVOT gradients.

Coronary angiography is required to assess suitable septal branches to the basal septum. Target septal arteries arise from coronary arteries other than the left anterior descending artery (LAD) in 15% of cases [18]. Coronary computerized tomographic angiography (CTA) has recently been described for the pre-procedural planning of an ASA scan for septal anatomy to help guide the selection of the target septal branch and is reportedly associated with a decreased need for ablation of other septal branches in small cohorts [19, 20].

Informed consent should be obtained as a shared decision-making process that begins before the procedure is scheduled. This involves a discussion on the disease mechanism, rationale for and alternatives to PTSMA as well as procedural risks and outcomes of all therapeutic options, being cognizant of the needs and preferences of the patient.

PROCEDURAL TECHNIQUES

INTRAPROCEDURAL IMAGING
Baseline imaging may be done with a trans-thoracic echocardiogram (TTE) or transesophageal echocardiogram (TEE). The decision of the best imaging depends on the expertise of the team and the comfort of the operator. Some operators elect to use TTE if the patient had excellent transthoracic imaging windows on prior imaging and LVOT gradient measures with a central aortic pressure and a retrograde left ventricular pigtail catheter. A TEE is preferred for the procedure because the basal septal and mitral valve is well visualized on mid-esophageal views. Additionally, TEE allows transeptal access for accurate intraprocedural hemodynamics to be safely guided; additional expertise of an imager is beneficial as part of a multidisciplinary heart team model.

ANESTHESIA
General anesthesia is needed for TEE imaging. If TTE is used, conscious sedation may be performed as long as adequate analgesia to tide the patient through the pain and discomfort of the iatrogenic infarct can be safely administered.

PACEMAKER
A temporary pacemaker is needed for back-up pacing if an intraprocedural or post-procedural atrioventricular block develops. The incidence of an atrioventricular block needing a permanent pacemaker is influenced by baseline conduction abnormalities and the alcohol dose. The area of infarction after PTSMA lies between the anterior two-thirds and the inferior one-third of the interventricular septum, where the right bundle lies [21]. A right bundle branch block occurs in approximately half of patients undergoing PTSMA. A complete atrioventricular block needing a pacemaker occurs in 10–15% of people with normal electrocardiograms at baseline. In patients with a baseline left-axis deviation, a left bundle branch block, or a wide QRS interval, the pacemaker requirement increases to 50%.

Balloon-tipped pacemakers can be used, though such use is associated with a risk of cardiac perforation, especially with long indwelling peri-procedural times due to stiffness. A low profile active fixation temporary pacemaker lead (e.g., Model 6416-140 Medtronic Inc. Fridley, MN) maintains a stable pacing, especially in the post-procedure period, allowing for reliable capture, and is associated with superior outcomes [22]. The pacemaker tip should be positioned away from the site of intended septal infarct to ensure continuous capture during PTSMA. If the patient has a permanent pacemaker in place prior to PTSMA, then pacing thresholds should be confirmed, especially if not pacemaker-dependent.

INVASIVE HEMODYNAMICS

A thorough invasive hemodynamic study should be performed before and after PTSMA to obtain gradients at rest and with provocation (e.g., premature ventricular beat, Valsalva, nitrates, isoproterenol). This is imperative because LVOT gradients post-PTSMA strongly predict long-term outcomes, including the need for repeat SRTs [14]. A retroaortic pigtail catheter is inserted into the ascending aorta from an arterial access. Transeptal catheterization is the best method for measuring LV pressures for the purpose of assessing LVOT gradients. Compared to retroaortic LV catheterization, transeptal LV catheterization avoids the risk of catheter entrapment, which can be difficult to distinguish from the very dynamic LV pressure changes that occur in HCM. Catheter entrapment results in falsely lowered gradients.

A sheath with a side port (e.g., Mullins or Agilis catheter, Abbott Vascular, Santa Clara, CA) is then inserted through the transeptal access into the left atrium (LA). A 7Fr balloon-tipped catheter with side holes (e.g., 7Fr Berman catheter, Arrow International Inc., Reading, PA) is inserted through this and steered into the left ventricle (LV). These allow for simultaneous LA and LV measurements for assessment of diastolic dysfunction associated with left ventricular hypertension and mitral regurgitation and to assess the impact of PTSMA on these.

For retroaortic LV pressures, a multipurpose catheter with side holes or a halo catheter should be used. A pigtail with side hole catheters is not useful because some or all of the holes may be positioned above the level of obstruction, causing falsely lowered gradients. End hole catheters are prone to entrapment. When using retroaortic LV pressure measurements, the absence of catheter entrapment may be excluded if there is pulsatile flow from the end of the catheter when it is disconnected from the pressure tubings. Alternatively, hand contrast injections through the catheter can show if there is an entrapment.

CORONARY ANGIOGRAPHY

After baseline hemodynamics have been obtained, the guide catheter is engaged in the parent artery of the septal artery to the basal septum on pre-procedure coronary angiograms or coronary CTA and reference angiograms are taken. While this is often from the proximal LAD, the target septal branch may arise from other branches, including the proximal right coronary artery (RCA) or conus branches, left circumflex, obtuse marginal, or left main coronary artery. The reference angiograms are observed carefully for contrast washout that may indicate that there is communication of the target septal with the posterior descending branch supplying the inferior third of the septum. At the same time, the angiograms should be assessed for other septal branches supplying the base of the septum which may become the target septal if additional LVOT gradient reduction is needed. The right anterior oblique (RAO) projections help outline the angulation of the target septal, left anterior oblique (LAO) projections help show the course of the septal at the basal septum, and cranial (CRA) projections help in assessing the length of the vessel. Factors for choosing a target septal are proximity to basal septum, width, and angulation. The length of the septal is less important because, while a septal branch may appear short, it can be wired distally for support. The RAO CRA view is a good working view as the length of the septal can be well visualized.

An ideal septal branch may not be identified in up to 10–20% of cases because of the concomitant supply of myocardium beyond the basal septum or because the size for interventional equipment [is too small (23, 24)].

PERCUTANEOUS TRANSLUMINAL SEPTAL MYOCARDIAL ABLATION OR ALCOHOL SEPTAL ABLATION

Conventional 6F or 7F catheters are used to engage the parent vessel of the target septal branch. This should be well seated and coaxial to allow good contrast opacification of the septal. Anticoagulation is given at the standard dose for percutaneous coronary interventions. The target septal branch is wired with a 0.014" guidewire – a moderate support workhorse wire with a floppy reshapable tip is suitable. In very angulated septal branches where wiring is difficult, an angled 0.014" microcatheter – such as a Twin-Pass dual access catheter, a SuperCross, or a

Venture catheter (all Teleflex Inc. Plymouth, MN) – may be needed for the target septal branch. The septal should be wired distally to allow tracking of the balloon into the septal and to ensure stable positioning of the interventional equipment during alcohol injection. After wiring, an over-the-wire (OTW) balloon is advanced to the proximal part of the septal. A slightly over-sized (1.3,1), short (6–12 mm) balloon is used. Balloon oversizing allows occlusion of the vessel at low pressures (3–4 atm), which in turn permits injection through the lumen of the OTW balloon with minimal risk of over-distension and vessel trauma or dissection.

After the balloon is inflated in the proximal target septal branch, well away from the parent branch, the wire is withdrawn, confirming on fluoroscopy that the balloon has not moved. Coronary angiography is repeated in the RAO projection to ensure that there is no communication between the occluded septal and the parent branch. Using a 3 cc syringe, undiluted radiographic contrast is gently injected through the inflated OTW balloon to perform selective angiography of the target septal. The injection should be gentle because if forceful it can cause vessel injury or undesirable opening of collaterals of unclear significance. This selective septal angiogram shows the length of the target septal and serves as a visualization of the path of the absolute alcohol when it is injected. The selective septal angiogram is examined to ensure that the balloon is well positioned, stable, the septal is completely occluded without leaks back to the parent vessel, and there is no contrast washout, that is, collaterals to the RCA or other vessels.

After this, through a 3 cc syringe, echo contrast is injected through the same OTW balloon under echocardiographic guidance. Any of the commercially available echo contrast agents can be used (e.g., Definity [Perflutren Lipid Microspheres], Lantheus Medical Imaging Billerica, MA; Optison [Perflutren Protein Type A microspheres] General Electric Company, CT; Lumason [sulfur hexafluoride lipid-type A microspheres], Bracco Diagnostics Inc., Monroe Township, NJ). The echo contrast should be diluted with saline to optimize myocardial opacification and minimize attenuation. The echocontrast should be injected slowly. Fast injections causes the echo contrast to fill the left ventricular cavity and may limit visualization. The echocardiogram is assessed to ensure that the target infarct area is the area of maximum flow acceleration in the LVOT in the area of SAM–septal contact. Other areas should be assessed to ensure that the non-target myocardium is not enhanced by echo contrast, especially the RV, papillary muscles, inferior wall, and anterior wall.

The desiccated (absolute) alcohol should not be placed on the procedure table because its contact with other objects can cause sclerosing of other tissues when in contact with them. The alcohol is withdrawn into a 3 cc syringe. The total amount to be injected is approximately 0.8–1.0 cc per cm of basal septal thickness [25]. A high volume of injection is associated with increased mortality [8]. The alcohol injection should be slow (~ 0.7–1.0 cc per min). If the injection is too fast there is a risk of atrioventricular (AV) block; if it is too slow, there is a risk of recanalization from wash out. The alcohol injection should be done under fluoroscopy to confirm a stable balloon position. After injection is completed, discard the syringe and flush the balloon lumen tubing with 1–2 cc saline via a 3 cc syringe.

Desiccated (absolute) alcohol is preferred for ablation because this agent immediately results in a discrete myocardial infarction. Other percutaneous methods of inducing a myocardial infarct (e.g., vascular coiling, covered stents) may slow down the flow but not result in immediate infarction. With a slow flow, there is a risk of opening and the development of septal collateralization, which prevents the infarction needed for effective septal ablation and LVOT gradient reduction.

The balloon should be left inflated for five to ten minutes after the alcohol has been flushed with saline to reduce the risk of alcohol extravasation into the parent vessel on withdrawal. Under fluoroscopy, the balloon is deflated and removed. The guide should be allowed to bleed back to ensure there is no residual alcohol before making any further injections through the guide.

Final coronary angiograms should show no flow or only slow flow through the injected septal branch. Also the parent vessel should be inspected for dissections or spasm. Final gradients should be assessed (Figure 12.1). The invasive hemodynamics should be done with the

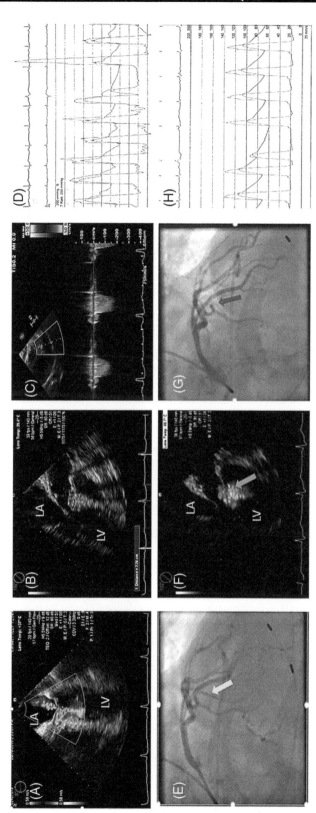

Figure 12.1 (A) A 68-year-old man with HCM. Symptoms are refractory to medical therapy. Baseline TEE shows flow acceleration in the LVOT and posteriorly directed mitral regurgitation due to SAM of the mitral valve. (B) Septal wall thickness measured at 2.26 cm. (C) Modest LVOT gradients on TEE of 16 mm Hg. (D) Invasive hemodynamics, LVOT gradients at rest of 20 mm Hg, and post-premature ventricular contraction > 140 mm Hg. (E) Target septal on angiogram (yellow arrow). (F) Basal septum highlighted after selective injection of echo contrast into basal septum. (G) No flow through target septal (red arrow) after PTSMA with 2 cc of alcohol. (H) After PTSMA, LVOT gradient at rest is 30 mm Hg and 40 mm Hg post-PVC.

interventional equipment withdrawn from the guide to prevent pressure dampening of wave-forms and underestimation of residual gradients. Procedural success is defined as a decrease in gradient to < 10 mm Hg at rest or a > 50% decrease in provocable gradients [14, 26]. An immediate residual gradient > 25 mm Hg predicts procedural failure. If the post-procedural gradients are not satisfactory, the procedure can be repeated through another septal. Before injecting another bolus of alcohol, collaterals which tend to be recruited after prolonged balloon inflation should be excluded with a septal angiography [27].

Post-procedure, the temporary pacemaker should be left for 48–72 hours and a permanent one placed if atrioventricular block ensues. A TTE in the days following the PTSMA may demonstrate elevated gradients due to edema associated with infarction, which should resolve over time.

COMPLICATIONS OF PERCUTANEOUS TRANSLUMINAL SEPTAL MYOCARDIAL ABLATION

The complications of PTSMA include systemic embolization, arrhythmias, coronary perforation, spasm, and dissections that occur with any percutaneous coronary intervention. Complications that are specific to ASA include non-target myocardial infarction, cardiac tamponade, papillary muscle infarct causing mitral regurgitation, ventricular septal defect, ventricular arrhythmias, sudden cardiac death, and atrioventricular block [26, 28, 29]. Peri-procedural mortality for ASA in contemporary experience is 0.7–1.0% [8, 30]. Specific complications to ASA that will be discussed further are early complications of non-target remote myocardial infarction, high grade AV block, early and late complications of ventricular arrhythmias, and the need for repeat interventions.

The peri-procedural complications may manifest > 48 hours after ASA, therefore these patients should be observed for at least 72 hours in at least an intermediate care unit.

Non-target remote myocardial infarction may be caused by egress of alcohol into the parent branch or through collaterals to the right coronary artery territory via its right posterior descending artery branch. Extravasation of alcohol into the parent branch through leakage around the balloon, the balloon slipping during alcohol injection, and poor balloon removal methods are known complications and care should be taken to avoid them. Attention to fluoroscopy, echocardiograms, and meticulous technique prevents most if not all of these complications. Where there are collaterals between the target septal branch and the right posterior descending artery (RPDA), ASA may still be performed by experienced operators if there are no other SRT alternatives. The technique described to overcome this involves engaging the RCA with another guide and a 0.014" wire passed to the collateralized RCA branch, often the RPDA. This branch is then occluded with a coronary balloon after which alcohol can be injected into the target septal, avoiding washout into the occluded RPDA collaterals, though with the risk of non-target myocardial infarction [31].

High grade atrioventricular block is reported to occur in approximately 10% of cases after ASA [8, 30, 32]. The rates are higher for initial experience, up to 30% [22]. This may be due to the fact that with earlier PTSMA experience high volumes of alcohol were the norm (average 4–5 cc). A complete AV block can happen during the procedure or more than 24 hours after it [33]. In a study of 31 consecutive ASA patients, 55% had intraprocedural AV block, 41% were resolved at the end of the procedure, and 65% of all the initial AV blocks were resolved within three days [34]. Conduction abnormalities occur because the target septal branch supplies the area of the septum where the right bundle branch is located, therefore infarct in this area causes a right bundle branch block. This has been demonstrated on cardiac MRI images which also show that myectomy results in a left bundle branch block because the area of excised muscle in myectomy is intimately related to the left bundle [21]. The factors that predict pacemaker dependency after PTSMA are age, baseline left bundle branch block, and high alcohol dose.

Ventricular arrhythmias have been reported to occur during PTSMA: early peri-procedural ventricular arrhythmia rates are ~ 1.6% [8, 26]. Long term, the impact of the post-PTSMA infarct scar on arrhythmia generation has been controversial. In two different cohorts of patients, postprocedure PTSMA has not been associated with a higher risk of ventricular arrhythmias in HCM patients [35, 36]. However, in another cohort comparing PTSMA and myectomy, up to a five-fold increase in death and appropriate defibrillator shocks were noted in the PTSMA patients. It should be noted that the first 25 of the 91 PTSMA procedures were done with up to 4.5 cc of alcohol, which is associated with worse outcomes and complications [16]. When compared to studies where the average alcohol dose was lower (< 2 cc), sudden cardiac death is low [14].

CLINICAL OUTCOMES OF PERCUTANEOUS TRANSLUMINAL SEPTAL MYOCARDIAL ABLATION

The primary goal of PTSMA is to achieve symptom relief with the least complications and without impairment of survival.

ACUTE PROCEDURAL SUCCESS
Acute procedural success, similar to myectomy, defined as ≥ 80% reduction in LVOT gradients at rest or with provocation, with a residual final resting gradient ≤ 10 mm Hg, occurs in 80–85% of patients undergoing PTSMA [14, 37].

Institutional and operator experience is pivotal to PTSMA success; a case volume of > 50 patients has been shown to be an independent predictor of survival, free of symptoms [28, 38]. The diameter of the parent LAD vessel > 4.0 cm and septal hypertrophy ≥ 18 mm is associated with poorer outcomes. A baseline LVOT gradient > 100 mm Hg is associated with reduced PTSMA success but has no impact on myomectomy success [37]. Age > 65 years is associated with greater symptom improvement with ASA.

When assessing LVOT gradients after PTSMA, it is important to note that the elevated gradients and LVOTO may be noted in the first few days post-procedure due to myocardial edema accompanying infarction, which resolves over time with ventricular remodeling. Thus, repeat TTE during the hospitalization after the procedure is not of benefit, unless there is a concern of complications. Ventricular remodeling at the site of infarction and also from the interventricular septum leads to continued reduction in LVOT gradients over three to six months.

Procedural failure or gradient reduction of < 50% or to > 25 mm Hg is most often a consequence of PTSMA through an inappropriate septal branch. An appropriate target septal is absent in 10–20% of cases [23, 24]. A higher residual gradient is associated with suboptimal symptom relief, increased risk of arrhythmias, and mortality in long-term follow-up. The need for repeat interventions occurs in ~5–10% of cases [26, 39, 40].

SYMPTOM RELIEF
The positive impact of PTSMA on functional class and exercise capacity has been described and shown to be directly related to the degree of LVOT gradient reduction [41]. The need for repeat interventions occurs in 5–10% of cases [26, 39, 40].

Some technical reasons for the need for repeat interventions are echocardiographic imaging challenges posed by shadowing from echocardiographic contrast limiting visualization of the basal septum from apical windows. This erroneously gives the impression that the ablation is adequate, leading to residual LVOTO in follow-up. Additionally balloon occlusion of the septal causes ischemia of the basal septum and myocardial stunning, showing reduced LVOT gradients during the procedure, though this is not sustained in follow-up.

Although clinical improvement with PTSMA is similar to myectomy in long-term studies, there is greater symptom relief when myectomy is performed in younger patients. This may be due to the fact that residual gradients after PTSMA are higher (10–20 mm Hg) compared to myectomy (< 10 mm Hg) and that higher gradients are less tolerable in younger active people.

SURVIVAL

A well-conducted randomized controlled trial will provide much information between PTSMA and myectomy and guide therapeutic decisions. Unfortunately, the frequency of needing SRTs poses practical limitations to such a trial [42]. Given these constraints, the best evidence for PTSMA comes from single-center cohort, multi-center registries, and properly performed meta-analyses of these patients.

The first study evaluating outcomes between PTSMA and myectomy in the United States looked at 177 patients in each arm [14]. The eight-year survival in the PTSMA group was identical to survival in myectomy patients in age- and gender-matched controls (79% for all three groups). Survival free of symptoms and the need for additional SRT at the eight-year follow-up in the PTSMA patients were 69.8% (60.9–78.8%) and 78.9% in myectomy patients (71.2–86.6%; P = 0.04). For the combined endpoint of sudden death and appropriate defibrillator discharge, the incidence in the PTSMA group was 1.41% (0.67–2.52%). Average alcohol volume in this study was 1.8 cc. Irrespective of SRT, the residual LVOT gradient ≥ 10 mm Hg was associated with decreased survival. This is likely a reflection of the complexity of HCM than the procedure itself.

Another study selected by a 2:1 propensity score, matching a cohort of 344 myectomy and 167 ASA patients, from patients who had undergone SRT at a single institution between 1998 and 2016. This showed no difference in peri-procedural complications, survival, or symptom relief in follow-up. There was a higher pacemaker requirement (3.9% vs. 17.4%, P < 0.001) and a need for repeat interventions in the ASA group (hazard ratio, 33.25; 95% confidence interval, 4.41–250.57; P < 0.001). Hospital stay was twice as long with myectomy (6.0 [5.0–7.0] days vs. 3.0 [3.0–4.0] days, P < 0.001) [43].

A multi-center North America study of 874 patients showed significant improvement with PTSMA: 95% improved to NYHA I-II, procedural mortality was < 0.7%, survival at 1, 5, and 9 years was 97%, 86%, and 74% respectively. Predictors of mortality during follow-up are a lower baseline left ventricular ejection fraction (LVEF), larger number of ablation procedures, and higher septal thickness [26].

The largest multinational PTSMA registry with long-term follow-up, the Euro-ASA registry, included over 1,200 patients who underwent PTSMA in ten institutions in seven countries from January 1996 to February 2015 [30]. This study provided invaluable insight into acute and long-term outcomes of PTSMA. The mean age of the patients was 58 ± 14 years, and the median ten-year survival was 77% (IQR 73–80%), consistent with safety and durability. Mortality and pacemaker requirements increased with increasing age after PTSMA, being lowest in patients ≤ 50 years (0.3% and 1% respectively) and ≥ 65 years (2% and 5% respectively) [44]. PTSMA was also found to be effective and safe in patients with only mild symptoms [45]. A subset of this registry from three centers studying young patients ≤ 50 years old with a median follow-up of five years (0.1–15.4 years), showed a low rate of mortality and an appropriate ICD discharge (1.43%; 95% CI, 0.52–3.10%) [46]. Another cohort from this registry generated, via propensity score matching, 172 pairs of patients with an interventricular septum (IVS) ≤ 16 mm and >16 mm, which was also followed up for 5.4 ± 4.3 years. There was no difference in symptom relief or LVOT gradient reduction between both groups. The patients with IVS ≤ 16 mm experienced higher early post-procedure complications (16% vs. 9%; P = 0.049) driven by higher pacemaker requirements in the IVS ≤ 16 mm group (13% vs. 8%; P = 0.22). There, patients with mild hypertrophy (IVS ≤ 16 mm) had fewer repeat interventions and no ventricular septal defect [47]. The annual mortality post-PTSMA in the registry was 2.4%. The risk of sudden cardiac death was 1% per year. Higher residual gradients were associated with poor outcomes. Although higher doses of alcohol were associated with more effective LVOT gradient reduction, this came at the price of an increased risk of pacemaker requirements. An average alcohol dose of 1.5–2.5 cc was found to be adequate to strike the balance between safety and efficacy [30]. An institutional experience of 50 or more procedures in the Euro-ASA registry was demonstrated to be associated with low complications, better symptom and gradient relief, and less need for repeat interventions [38].

Several meta-analyses have compared PTSMA and myectomy [39, 40, 48, 49]. The largest included a PTSMA cohort (n = 4,213; follow-up = 6.6 years) and a myectomy cohort (n = 4,240; follow-up = 6.8 years) [40]. This showed a higher peri-procedural mortality and stroke in the myectomy group (2.0% vs. 1.2%, P = 0.009 and 1.5% vs. 0.8%, P = 0.013, respectively). The PTSMA group had a higher rate of pacemaker implantation (10% vs. 5%, P < 0.001). Between the PTSMA and myectomy cohorts, there was no difference in all-cause death (1.5% vs. 1.1% per person year, P = 0.21 respectively), cardiovascular death (0.4% vs. 0.5% per person year, P = 0.53), and sudden cardiac death (0.3% vs. 0.3% per person year, P = 0.43). The need for repeat intervention was higher in the PTSMA group (11% vs. 1.5%, P < 0.001).

OTHER PERCUTANEOUS SEPTAL ABLATION METHODS

Percutaneous radio frequency (RF) ablation of the interventricular septum has also been described for the relief of LVOTO. This technique uses RF to ablate the septal myocardium from an endocardial approach without the constraints of septal anatomy and reliance on large septal infarct for LVOT gradient reduction. Initial experience was performed with RF needles passed via retroaortic, transmitral, or via right ventricle approaches into the LVOT. This was associated with higher residual gradients leading to hesitancy with this approach [50]. More recently a newer technique for percutaneous RF ablation in HCM was described, namely percutaneous intramyocardial biopsy multi-range ablation (PIMSRA) [51]. This procedure is performed via transapical access. The RF needle is passed via ultrasound-guided apical access into the myocardium of the interventricular septum. When the end of the needle is positioned at base of the septum, ~ 10 mm from the subaortic membranous septum, the ablation power is increased gradually from 60 W to 140 W and applied for ≤ 12 minutes. This is done under continuous EKG monitoring. The ablation is terminated if there is ST elevation. The goal of the procedure is hemodynamic relief or evidence of necrosis on a contrast enhanced echocardiogram. The initial small report showed excellent LVOT gradient reduction in 15 patients without mortality or pacemaker reduction. The long-term effect of a mid-wall scar on systolic and diastolic function as well as future arrhythmias is unclear.

HYPERTROPHIC CARDIOMYOPATHY HEART TEAMS AND CENTERS

The heart team model has been beneficial in decision making regarding therapeutic options in valves, coronary artery disease, and advanced heart failure therapies. A similar model for HCM should be tasked with decision making regarding the best therapeutic options for SRTs, arrhythmia management, advanced heart failure therapies, research participation, and improvement of quality metrics in the care of HCM patients. This team should include a clinical cardiologist, a multimodality imaging cardiologist, a cardiac surgeon, an interventional cardiologist experienced in septal reduction therapies, an electrophysiologist, and heart failure/cardiomyopathy specialists.

The outcome of SRT has clearly been demonstrated to be best when care is delivered at centers with the highest level of experience [6, 7, 28, 38, 52].

CONCLUSION

The data limitations posed by the lack of randomized controlled trials continues to fuel the debates regarding which SRT is superior. The residual LVOT gradient is consistently associated with worse outcomes, therefore elimination of this gradient is a more important consideration than the method, as long as the chosen SRT can be safely performed with the least complications [47]. Over the past three decades, with increasing experience, PTSMA has evolved to use more refined imaging guidance and infarct localization with echo contrast and reduced alcohol volume. The earlier concern about the arrhythmogenicity of myocardial scarring appears to be unfounded with contemporary PTSMA techniques [35, 36]. Therefore PTSMA has emerged as an invaluable, accessible technique for the management of symptoms attributable to drug-refractory HCM in appropriately selected patients. With accumulating long-term follow-up retrospective data, pacemaker requirement, and reintervention for symptomatic LVOT, gradients remain the only outcomes where myectomy performs better than PTSMA.

In the absence of randomized controlled data, mandatory reporting akin to those established for surgical and transcatheter valve interventions will facilitate registry data from which meaningful long-term data on patient selection and optimization of outcomes can be derived.

REFERENCES

1. Maron BJ, Gardin JM, Flack JM, Gidding SS, Kurosaki TT, Bild DE. Prevalence of hypertrophic cardiomyopathy in a general population of young adults: echocardiographic analysis of 4111 subjects in the CARDIA Study–Coronary Artery Risk Development in (Young) Adults. *Circulation* 1995;92:785–789.
2. Semsarian C, Ingles J, Maron MS, Maron BJ. New perspectives on the prevalence of hypertrophic cardiomyopathy. *J. Am. Coll. Cardiol.* 2015;65:1249–1254.
3. Maron BJ. Clinical course and management of hypertrophic cardiomyopathy. *N. Engl. J. Med.* 2018;379:1977.
4. Sigwart U. Non-surgical myocardial reduction for hypertrophic obstructive cardiomyopathy. *Lancet* 1995;346:211–214.
5. Morrow AG, Reitz BA, Epstein SE, et al. Operative treatment in hypertrophic subaortic stenosis: techniques, and the results of pre and postoperative assessments in 83 patients. *Circulation* 1975;52:88–102.
6. Maron BJ, Dearani JA, Ommen SR, et al. Low operative mortality achieved with surgical septal myectomy: role of dedicated hypertrophic cardiomyopathy centers in the management of dynamic subaortic obstruction. *J. Am. Coll. Cardiol.* 2015;66:1307–1308.
7. Kim LK, Swaminathan RV, Looser P, et al. Hospital volume outcomes after septal myectomy and alcohol septal ablation for treatment of obstructive hypertrophic cardiomyopathy: US nationwide inpatient database, 2003–2011. *JAMA Cardiol.* 2016;1:324–332.
8. Nagueh SF, Groves BM, Schwartz L, et al. Alcohol septal ablation for the treatment of hypertrophic obstructive cardiomyopathy. A multicenter North American registry. *J. Am. Coll. Cardiol.* 2011;58:2322–2328.
9. Panaich SS, Badheka AO, Chothani A, et al. Results of ventricular septal myectomy and hypertrophic cardiomyopathy (from Nationwide Inpatient Sample [1998–2010]). *Am. J. Cardiol.* 2014;114:1390–1395.
10. Ommen SR, Nishimura RA. Hypertrophic cardiomyopathy-one case per year? A clarion call to do what is right. *JAMA Cardiol.* 2016;1:333–334.

11. Elliott PM, Anastasakis A, et al. 2014 ESC guidelines on diagnosis and management of hypertrophic cardiomyopathy: the Task Force for the Diagnosis and Management of Hypertrophic Cardiomyopathy of the European Society of Cardiology (ESC). *Eur. Heart J.* 2014;35:2733–2779.

12. Gersh BJ, Maron BJ, Bonow RO, et al. 2011 ACCF/AHA guideline for the diagnosis and treatment of hypertrophic cardiomyopathy: a report of the American College of Cardiology Foundation/American Heart Association Task Force on Practice Guidelines–developed in collaboration with the American Association for Thoracic Surgery, American Society of Echocardiography, American Society of Nuclear Cardiology, Heart Failure Society of America, Heart Rhythm Society, Society for Cardiovascular Angiography and Interventions, and Society of Thoracic Surgeons. *J. Am. Coll. Cardiol.* 2011;58:e212–e260.

13. Maron BJ, Yacoub M, Dearani JA. Controversies in cardiovascular medicine. Benefits of surgery in obstructive hypertrophic cardiomyopathy: bring septal myectomy back for European patients. *Eur. Heart J.* 2011;32:1055–1058.

14. Sorajja P, Ommen SR, Holmes DR, et al. Survival after alcohol septal ablation for obstructive hypertrophic cardiomyopathy. *Circulation* 2012;126:2374–2380.

15. Sorajja P, Pedersen WA, Bae R, et al. First experience with percutaneous mitral valve plication as primary therapy for symptomatic obstructive hypertrophic cardiomyopathy. *J. Am. Coll. Cardiol.* 2016;67:2811–2818.

16. ten Cate FJ, Soliman OII, Michels M, et al. Long-term outcome of alcohol septal ablation in patients with obstructive hypertrophic cardiomyopathy: a word of caution. *Circ. Heart Fail.* 2010;3:362–369.

17. Veselka J, Jensen M, Liebregts M, et al. Alcohol septal ablation in patients with severe septal hypertrophy. *Heart* 2020;106:462–466.

18. Alkhouli M, Sajjad W, Lee J, et al. Prevalence of non-left anterior descending septal perforator culprit in patients with hypertrophic cardiomyopathy undergoing alcohol septal ablation. *Am. J. Cardiol.* 2016;117:1655–1660.

19. Cooper RM, Binukrishnan SR, Shahzad A, Hasleton J, Sigwart U, Stables RH. Computed tomography angiography planning identifies the target vessel for optimum infarct location and improves clinical outcome in alcohol septal ablation for hypertrophic obstructive cardiomyopathy. *Euro. Intervention* 2017;12:e2194–e2203.

20. Yanagiuchi T, Tada N, Haga Y, et al. Utility of preprocedural multidetector computed tomography in alcohol septal ablation for hypertrophic obstructive cardiomyopathy. *Cardiovasc. Interv. Ther.* 2019;34:364–372.

21. Valeti US, Nishimura RA, Holmes DR, et al. Comparison of surgical septal myectomy and alcohol septal ablation with cardiac magnetic resonance imaging in patients with hypertrophic obstructive cardiomyopathy. *J. Am. Coll. Cardiol.* 2007;49:350–357.

22. Talreja DR, Nishimura RA, Edwards WD, et al. Alcohol septal ablation versus surgical septal myectomy: comparison of effects on atrioventricular conduction tissue. *J. Am. Coll. Cardiol.* 2004;44:2329–2332.

23. Angelini P. The "1st septal unit" in hypertrophic obstructive cardiomyopathy: a newly recognized anatomo-functional entity, identified during recent alcohol septal ablation experience. *Tex. Heart Inst. J.* 2007;34:336–346.

24. Singh M, Edwards WD, Holmes DR, Tajil AJ, Nishimura RA. Anatomy of the first septal perforating artery: a study with implications for ablation therapy for hypertrophic cardiomyopathy. *Mayo Clin. Proc.* 2001;76:799–802.

25. Faber L, Seggewiss H, Welge D, et al. Echo-guided percutaneous septal ablation for symptomatic hypertrophic obstructive cardiomyopathy: 7 years of experience. *Eur. J. Echocardiogr.* 2004;5:347–355.

26. Nagueh SF, Bierig SM, Budoff MJ, et al. American Society of Echocardiography clinical recommendations for multimodality cardiovascular imaging of patients with hypertrophic cardiomyopathy: endorsed by the American Society of Nuclear Cardiology, Society for Cardiovascular Magnetic Resonance, and Society of Cardiovascular Computed Tomography. *J. Am. Soc. Echocardiogr.* 2011;24:473–498.

27. Rigopoulos A, Sepp R, Palinkas A, Ungi I, Kremastinos DT, Seggewiss H. Alcohol septal ablation for hypertrophic obstructive cardiomyopathy: collateral vessel communication between septal branches. *Int. J. Cardiol.* 2006;113:e67-e69.
28. Sorajja P, Binder J, Nishimura RA, et al. Predictors of an optimal clinical outcome with alcohol septal ablation for obstructive hypertrophic cardiomyopathy. *Catheter Cardiovasc. Interv.* 2013;81:E58-E67.
29. Alam M, Dokainish H, Lakkis N. Alcohol septal ablation for hypertrophic obstructive cardiomyopathy: a systematic review of published studies. *J. Interv. Cardiol.* 2006;19:319–327.
30. Veselka J, Jensen MK, Liebregts M, et al. Long-term clinical outcome after alcohol septal ablation for obstructive hypertrophic cardiomyopathy: results from the Euro-ASA registry. *Eur. Heart J.* 2016;37:1517–1523.
31. Koljaja-Batzner A, Pfeiffer B, Seggewiss H. Septal collateralization to right coronary artery in alcohol septal ablation: solution to a dangerous pitfall. *JACC Cardiovasc. Interv.* 2018;11:2009–2011.
32. Batzner A, Pfeiffer B, Neugebauer A, Aicha D, Blank C, Seggewiss H. Survival after alcohol septal ablation in patients with hypertrophic obstructive cardiomyopathy. *J. Am. Coll. Cardiol.* 2018;72:3087–3094.
33. Veselka J, Lawrenz T, Stellbrink C, et al. Low incidence of procedure-related major adverse cardiac events after alcohol septal ablation for symptomatic hypertrophic obstructive cardiomyopathy. *Can. J. Cardiol.* 2013;29:1415–1421.
34. Reinhard W, Ten Cate FJ, Scholten M, De Laat LE, Vos J. Permanent pacing for complete atrioventricular block after nonsurgical (alcohol) septal reduction in patients with obstructive hypertrophic cardiomyopathy. *Am. J. Cardiol.* 2004;93:1064–1066.
35. Cuoco FA, Spencer WH, Fernandes VL, et al. Implantable cardioverter-defibrillator therapy for primary prevention of sudden death after alcohol septal ablation of hypertrophic cardiomyopathy. *J. Am. Coll. Cardiol.* 2008;52:1718–1723.
36. Jensen MK, Prinz C, Horstkotte D, et al. Alcohol septal ablation in patients with hypertrophic obstructive cardiomyopathy: low incidence of sudden cardiac death and reduced risk profile. *Heart* 2013;99:1012–1017.
37. Sorajja P, Valeti U, Nishimura RA, et al. Outcome of alcohol septal ablation for obstructive hypertrophic cardiomyopathy. *Circulation* 2008;118:131–139.
38. Veselka J, Faber L, Jensen MK, et al. Effect of institutional experience on outcomes of alcohol septal ablation for hypertrophic obstructive cardiomyopathy. *Can. J. Cardiol.* 2018;34:16–22.
39. Liebregts M, Vriesendorp PA, Mahmoodi BK, Schinkel AFL, Michels M, ten Berg JM. A systematic review and meta-analysis of long-term outcomes after septal reduction therapy in patients with hypertrophic cardiomyopathy. *JACC Heart Fail.* 2015;3:896–905.
40. Osman M, Kheiri B, Osman K, et al. Alcohol septal ablation vs myectomy for symptomatic hypertrophic obstructive cardiomyopathy: Systematic review and meta-analysis. *Clin. Cardiol.* 2019;42:190–197.
41. Fernandes VL, Nielsen C, Nagueh SF, et al. Follow-up of alcohol septal ablation for symptomatic hypertrophic obstructive cardiomyopathy the Baylor and Medical University of South Carolina experience 1996 to 2007. *JACC Cardiovasc. Interv.* 2008;1:561–570.
42. Olivotto I, Ommen SR, Maron MS, Cecchi F, Maron BJ. Surgical myectomy versus alcohol septal ablation for obstructive hypertrophic cardiomyopathy. Will there ever be a randomized trial? *J. Am. Coll. Cardiol.* 2007;50:831–834.
43. Nguyen A, Schaff HV, Hang D, et al. Surgical myectomy versus alcohol septal ablation for obstructive hypertrophic cardiomyopathy: a propensity score-matched cohort. *J. Thorac. Cardiovasc. Surg.* 2019;157:306-315.e3.
44. Liebregts M, Faber L, Jensen MK, et al. Outcomes of alcohol septal ablation in younger patients with obstructive hypertrophic cardiomyopathy. *JACC Cardiovasc. Interv.* 2017;10:1134–1143.

45. Veselka J, Faber L, Liebregts M, et al. Outcome of alcohol septal ablation in mildly symptomatic patients with hypertrophic obstructive cardiomyopathy: a long-term follow-up study based on the euro-alcohol septal ablation registry. *J. Am. Heart Assoc.* 2017;6.

46. Veselka J, Krejčí J, Tomašov P, et al. Survival of patients ≤ 50 years of age after alcohol septal ablation for hypertrophic obstructive cardiomyopathy. *Can. J. Cardiol.* 2014;30:634–638.

47. Veselka J, Faber L, Liebregts M, et al. Short- and long-term outcomes of alcohol septal ablation for hypertrophic obstructive cardiomyopathy in patients with mild left ventricular hypertrophy: a propensity score matching analysis. *Eur. Heart J.* 2019;40:1681–1687.

48. Agarwal S, Tuzcu EM, Desai MY, et al. Updated meta-analysis of septal alcohol ablation versus myectomy for hypertrophic cardiomyopathy. *J. Am. Coll. Cardiol.* 2010;55:823–834.

49. Leonardi RA, Kransdorf EP, Simel DL, Wang A. Meta-analyses of septal reduction therapies for obstructive hypertrophic cardiomyopathy: comparative rates of overall mortality and sudden cardiac death after treatment. *Circ. Cardiovasc. Interv.* 2010;3:97–104.

50. Sorajja P, Katsiyiannis WT, Harris KM. Searching for surgical alternatives in hypertrophic cardiomyopathy. *J. Am. Coll. Cardiol.* 2018;72:1910–1912.

51. Liu L, Li J, Zuo L, et al. Percutaneous intramyocardial septal radiofrequency ablation for hypertrophic obstructive cardiomyopathy. *J. Am. Coll. Cardiol.* 2018;72:1898–1909.

52. van der Lee C, Scholzel B, ten Berg JM, et al. Usefulness of clinical, echocardiographic, and procedural characteristics to predict outcome after percutaneous transluminal septal myocardial ablation. *Am. J. Cardiol.* 2008;101:1315–1320.

INDEX